ABORTING
PLANNED
PARENTHOOD

ABORTING PLANNED PARENTHOOD

Robert H. Ruff

LIFE CYCLE BOOKS LTD.
Toronto, Ontario • Lewiston, New York

First Printing, August, 1988
Second Printing, November, 1988
Third Printing, April, 1990

Published by:

Life Cycle Books Ltd.
2205 Danforth Avenue
Toronto, Ontario
M4C 1K4
(416) 690-5860

Printed in the U.S.A.

U.S.A. office:
Life Cycle Books
P.O. Box 420
Lewiston, NY 14092-0420

ISBN 0-919225-32-2

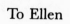
To Ellen

CONTENTS

ACKNOWLEDGMENTS

Without the generosity and hands-on help of many friends, this book would not have been possible.

I'd especially like to thank my parents, who provided the necessary capital for this project along with some useful words of wisdom.

The Larkin family also provided much encouragement and exhortation to help hold the project together.

Matthew Jackson played a crucial role in helping to gather the actual Planned Parenthood internal records, without which this book could not have been written.

Kathe Salazar, Karen Hartman, Karen Chakerian, Nina Neisig, and many others spent hundreds of hours inputting data into databases and typing manuscripts, while Lynn Hawley's copyediting strengthened the cohesiveness of the text and brought uniformity to the style.

Margaret Hotze of Life Advocates in Houston, Texas, provided many introductions to invaluable political and governmental sources in Washington, D.C., and was instrumental in the production of the book. Author George Grant supplied valuable advice regarding content and tone.

To each of you, my warmest thanks and best wishes.

When the solutions are the problem,
you've really got a problem.

PART ONE

THE PROBLEM

ONE

ABORTING PLANNED PARENTHOOD: GETTING THE FACTS

Matthew was frantically trying to pull something heavy out of the dumpster. We had been searching Planned Parenthood's huge dumpster for weeks, looking for dead babies, and so far we had not found any.

We had found the usual evidence of first trimester abortions: the medical bags stuffed with bloody medical gowns, blood-soaked gauze sheets, long clear suction tubes still coated internally with blood, slender cannulas with bits of bloody flesh still clinging to them, empty syringes, splattered discarded urine samples, and the ever-present, sickening smell of alcohol and blood and urine mingled together into an oppressive stench of death.

But no babies.

We simply could not figure out what they were doing with the babies. We wondered if they were pouring them down the sink (suction-aborted babies rarely need a disposal) or maybe flushing them down the toilet. Still, we figured that sooner or later some dead babies were going to show up in that dumpster.

Usually, I would go to the clinic by myself, late at night, and quickly remove only the medical bags. (We soon learned to distinguish the medical bags from the bathroom trash bags or the lunchroom trash bags or the clerical staff's trash bags.) Then I would drive home and methodically empty and refill the bags, looking for babies.

Rummaging through all that blood and urine three times a week was really getting to be a drag, especially since we still had not found any babies. Day-by-day, the whole trash monitoring effort started to look pretty pointless. Besides, my neighbors were beginning to wonder how we managed to generate thirty-five bags of household trash for curb-side collection every Tuesday and Friday.

We had been picketing Planned Parenthood for over three years now, with some success—but always with more faith and hope than success and results.

About two years earlier, we had started preaching to supplement our picketing, literature distribution, and sidewalk counseling. We would hand out pro-life literature to the women entering the clinic, occasionally convincing one to stop and talk long enough to persuade her not to have the abortion. But once the women were all inside, we'd start the preaching—just simple Bible passages, hammering away for an hour or more.

The clinic hated us. Almost weekly, they reported us to the Houston police. Each week was a new adventure as we waited to see which officers would show up and what the new complaint would be. The officers' reactions ranged from sympathetic, to obnoxious, to hostile, but they never once made an arrest. Usually they would tell us to move or to keep quiet, or they would make up some nitpicking rule like "no signs leaning against the planter boxes," but we would always refuse to comply on "free speech" and "lawful assembly" grounds.

Not that the clinic didn't make us nervous. It did. People who kill babies don't exactly respect adults' lives or civil rights, either.

The clinic employed a security guard full time and had installed an expensive halon gas fire suppression system; they were convinced that the clinic would be firebombed any day. At night, a security service conducted regular patrols.

That was the only problem with the dumpster raids. The dumpster was on the east side of the building, about seventy-five feet from the street, but it was situated directly underneath several extremely bright halogen lights. If the security service were to drive by and catch us in the dumpster, we'd be in trouble.

This night I had phoned my friend Matthew Jackson and asked him if he wouldn't mind coming along. Matthew was more than happy to help, and I was relieved to have some back-up along.

When we arrived at the clinic, we parked in the usual spot at an adjacent building and approached the dumpster. To my surprise, it was completely full, overflowing really, which was unusual anytime, but especially for a Tuesday night.

I had explained to Matthew how to identify the medical bags, and what our story would be if we were caught. And then, suddenly, there was Matthew on the other side of this huge dumpster with this strangely smug look on his face, frantically pulling something heavy from underneath some of the medical bags.

Whatever it was, he got it out and went right back to the same spot and started pulling something else out. This time I caught a better glimpse of it.

It was a computer printout.

I walked around the dumpster and began to examine what Matthew was removing, and it looked like we might be on to some important documents, financial records of some kind. Meanwhile, Matthew had returned to the dumpster and was throwing medical bags off the top.

We couldn't believe our eyes. The whole dumpster seemed to be stuffed to the brim with all kinds of file boxes, full of records. I jumped in and began to throw off the rest of the bags to see if it was just an illusion or if the dumpster really was full of boxes of clinic records.

It was full.

Still, it seemed too good to be true. Maybe there was really only a thin layer of records between two layers of trash. I began to dig down deep with my feet. No trashbags. Corrugated boxes. Papers.

Neither of us said a word—we both knew what to do. I went to fetch the car while Matthew extracted several big boxes of records. Quickly, we loaded up my station wagon one-foot deep with boxes of records and armfuls of loose folders full of records.

We started to load more when we remembered—the security patrol! Probably best to take this load home and then come back. It wouldn't do us any good to load up the whole car and then get caught by the security service and have to give it all back.

I drove as safely as you can at 85 MPH. We dumped the load in my garage and then I dropped Matthew by his house so he could bring his pickup truck. Matthew followed me back to the clinic, stopping along the way to peel off his several pro-life bumper stickers: no need to advertise trouble to the security patrol.

If we got caught by the security guards, we would tell them that we were just two small businessmen unloading some records into a spare dumpster. Our hope was that the security guards would then order us to remove all of the records from the dumpster.

When we arrived back at the clinic, we repeated our frantic loading process, with me in the dumpster handing armfuls of records to Matthew. It took two trips with both vehicles completely full to empty the dumpster. Well, actually, we left a few inches of records on the bottom.

Back at my garage, we began to sort the documents into stacks according to size and type of record. After a couple of hours' work, we could already make a pretty good rough estimate of what we had: tens of thousands of medical records, complete accounting and financial records, confidential internal memoranda, donor lists, a whole file box of actual abortion records (including employees' accounts of the horrifying complications during the abortions)—all-in-all, about two years' worth of the records of the nation's third largest Planned Parenthood affiliate.

A gold mine, in other words.

I immediately knew that, morally, we had to analyze these records and find out, for the first time ever, whether Planned Parenthood was really guilty of all the medical and financial scams of which it has always been accused.

In particular, the clinic visit records (CVRs) looked like a database waiting to happen. We had well over 50,000 CVRs, each one detailing dozens of pertinent items about a patient's visit. Each CVR contained complete demographic, medical, and billing information on a single patient. The possibilities were endless.

Database. We needed a computerized database. There was no way we could tabulate 50,000 CVRs by hand.

We bought three computers, programmed a database to receive every jot and tittle of the CVR information, trained several volunteers, and began inputting. And inputting.

And inputting. Six thousand records later, we quit. Six thousand records was a huge sample—plenty big for indisputably valid statistical analysis, but still small enough to be handled by one of our PCs.

What follows in this book are the results of thousands of hours of painstaking analysis of that database, a database that tells the story of a massive scam.

But this book is a lot more than just the factual, hard proof that Planned Parenthood really *is* raping taxpayers. It's a book about planned failure—the failure of birth control to prevent problem pregnancies and abortions, the failure of contraceptive-oriented sex education courses, the failure of "safe sex" (in theory and in clinic practice), and the failure of "safe, legal" abortions to make intrauterine infanticide safe.

Aborting Planned Parenthood does what no other book has ever done: It exposes the incredible scams, distortions, and failures of Planned Parenthood, using firsthand proof—actual confidential Planned Parenthood records and internal memos. No longer are the allegations of taxpayer rape and abuse merely informed hunches—now, for the first time ever, we have carefully researched and documented evidence provided by Planned Parenthood itself.

All of the evidence presented in this book comes from Planned Parenthood, the U.S. Government, or a pro-choice source; no pro-life sources are used. Names have been altered to protect the privacy of both the victims and the perpetrators of abortion.

The story told here is a story of tragedy. We find no pleasure in exposing the scandal and failure, because the victims are real—women and young girls, taxpayers, and families trying to raise their kids right. It's a sad story, but it's time someone told it.

T W O

THE TAXPAYER'S DAUGH-
TER: THE SCANDAL OF
GOVERNMENT FUNDING
OF PLANNED
PARENTHOOD

In a memo entitled "The Essential Facts on Family Planning
Funding Needs in Texas," Planned Parenthood of Houston and
Southeast Texas claimed that a projected $400,000 decrease in state
family planning funds would be disastrous for the state budget:

If this decrease occurs, Texas can absolutely count on

- more births to indigent women;
- a higher welfare caseload;
- increased cases of child abuse;
- greater demand for subsidized health care services;
- greater demand for day care services;
- greater demand for public housing.

This is the standard blackmail rhetoric of the family plan-
ning/abortion industry: Shovel us the money we want, or you'll
drown in a sea of new welfare babies (*abused* welfare babies).

This argument is accepted as gospel by Planned Parenthood
and by most members of Congress.

But it's false, *absolutely* false.

The overriding thrust behind governmental financing of family
planning programs has always been the presumption that gov-

9

ernment expenditures for family planning actually save the government money by reducing the breeding of legions of indigents, and therefore decreasing welfare expenditures. The economic argument has been something to the effect that every dollar spent for family planning reduces government welfare expenditures by two to three dollars.

While seeking to reduce government dependency among the indigent, the federal government has created a new class of government dependents: family planning organizations and clinics, primarily Planned Parenthood.

Planned Parenthood likes to bill itself as America's largest and oldest privately funded, nonprofit family planning organization.[1] In reality, much of Planned Parenthood's funding, at whatever level — national, international, or local — comes from taxpayer funds, funds that are used to finance the nation's largest chain of abortuaries (approximately 100,000 abortions per year), to finance the dispensing of unsafe contraceptive methods to teen-agers without their parents' consent, and to lobby on local, state, and national levels for more government funding of Planned Parenthood.

Many people are aware that Planned Parenthood receives tens of millions of dollars in government funds through Title X of the Public Health Service Act. Federal appropriations for Title X were $142.5 million in fiscal 1987.

Title X funds are important to Planned Parenthood because they are dispensed as outright gifts to be used as the clinics see fit. Title X is the only program that pays directly for the establishment and maintenance of birth control clinics and abortuaries.[2]

But Title X funds do not compose the majority of governmental funding for Planned Parenthood. Planned Parenthood also manages to receive funding under Title V (the Maternal and Child Health program of the Social Security Act), Title XIX (Medicaid), and Title XX (the Social Services program under the Social Security Act). In 1982, for instance, the federal government spent at least $17 million for family planning under

---

1. Nonprofit does not mean unprofitable or charitable. Nonprofit merely means that dividends cannot be paid to owners. Nonprofit organizations are often very profitable.

2. Alan Guttmacher Institute, *Issues in Brief*, 4:1 (March, 1984).

Title V, $46 million under Title XX, and $94 million under Title XIX, in addition to $130 million under Title X.[3]

But the federal funding does not end there. In fiscal 1984, the Center for Population Research managed to spend $8 million for contraceptive development, $3 million for contraceptive evaluation, $66 million for "reproductive sciences," and $14 million for demographic and behavioral research.[4] The Center for Population Research is part of the National Institute for Child Health and Human Development, which is funded through the National Institutes of Health, which in turn is funded under the Department of Health and Human Services.

These figures pertain mainly to direct federal expenditures, and do not include much of what is spent at the state level or lower.

Because of changes enacted at the urging of the Reagan administration, much federal funding of Planned Parenthood and of other antifamily organizations is virtually impossible to trace. Prior to 1981, states who wanted to spend Title V or XX funds were required to submit a detailed spending proposal. In addition, the states were obligated to report back to the federal government on a regular basis how they spent the funds, and how effective those expenditures were.

Many conservatives, however, felt that the accountability requirements were counterproductive because they really provided states an excuse to request more funds. The states would report that they spent $100 million on family planning and that teen pregnancy rates rose another 10%: ergo, more federal funding was needed to combat teen pregnancy.

The solution proposed by the Reagan administration was to drop all state accountability for how the funds are spent. Most federal funds allocated for family planning are now given to the states as no-strings-attached gifts known as block grants, and the states are free to use these funds as they see fit. They can fund abortions directly, or they can contract with Planned Parenthood clinics to perform family planning services for the state. In addition, there are no federal requirements to establish eligibility guidelines; states are free to dispense the funds to anyone, rich or poor.

---

3. Ibid.
4. Ibid.

This change of policy has made it nearly impossible to accurately trace the full extent of federal funding of anti-family activities, including those of Planned Parenthood.

It is probably safe to estimate that Planned Parenthood clinics receive at least $50 million per year in direct government payments for patient services, plus $30 million from Title X.[5]

An analysis of confidential 1984 internal financial records of 145 Planned Parenthood affiliates reveals the following statistics:

1. Government funding provided an average of 40% of the affiliates' total revenues and up to 80% of total income for some affiliates.

2. Title X provided 48% of total government funding, while Titles V, XIX, XX, and other federal programs provided 40% and state and local governments provided 12%.

3. Government funding provided the majority of revenues at more than half of the affiliates.

FUNDING COMPOSITION OF 145 PLANNED PARENTHOOD AFFILIATES, 1984 DATA

Title X:	$24,386,081
Title XX:	9,437,646
Title V:	2,563,999
Title XIX:	6,442,061
Other Federal:	1,882,676
State Governmment:	4,527,867
Local Government:	1,250,568
Total Government:	$50,490,898
United Way:	1,828,892
Other Sources:	76,533,960
Total Income:	$128,853,750
Avg. % Govt. Funding:	40%

Government funding of these 145 affiliates totaled $50,490,000 in 1984. As there are about 200 total Planned Parenthood affiliates, we can extrapolate this figure to arrive at an estimated $69,641,000

---

5. These figures ignore uncounted tens of millions which flow to Planned Parenthood Federation of America, International Planned Parenthood Federation, Alan Guttmacher Institute, and other related organizations for programs other than direct U.S. clinic support and services.

in total government funding for Planned Parenthood clinics in 1984. This figure includes income of the affiliates only; it does not include government funding provided to Planned Parenthood Federation of America (PPFA) or any of its sister organizations.

Obviously, the commonly quoted $30 million figure for government funding of Planned Parenthood is far too low. Title X alone contributes at least $30 million, while other government programs contribute another $40 million, just at the clinic level.

Inventing the Poor

The funds expended annually by the federal government for family planning could pay for the distribution of five hundred condoms per year to every woman of reproductive age in the United States — which brings up an interesting question: Just how effective are those government expenditures at producing welfare savings?

Well, Planned Parenthood insists that 80% of the women who visit its clinics are economically disadvantaged or indigent and therefore in need of government funding. However, while it is true that taxpayers foot the bill for up to 80% of all client visits to Planned Parenthood clinics, it is not true that these clients are truly needy. *In fact, probably 90% to 95% of all non-Medicaid clients who receive government funding for a visit to a Planned Parenthood clinic are not needy and are both willing and able to pay for the visit.*

An analysis of six thousand randomly selected client visit records from Planned Parenthood of Houston and Southeast Texas (PPHSET) supports this conclusion. Client demographics were analyzed by the client's method of payment: cash, Title XX, or Title XIX (Medicaid).

DEMOGRAPHIC CHARACTERISTICS OF PPHSET CLIENTS, BY PAYMENT METHOD

Payment Method	Avg Age	Average Number of Dependents	% on Welfare	% Anglo	Ethnicity % Black	% Hispanic	% Divorced, Widowed, or Separated	% Divorced, Widowed, or Separated & Unemployed
Cash, Full-Rate	24	2.1	5	59	22	16	18	6.9
Cash, Reduced-Rate	23	1.9	< 1	68	15	16	15	3.1
Title XX	22	2.0	3	59	19	21	16	8.4
Title XIX (Medicaid)	**23**	**2.9**	**70**	**18**	**63**	**17**	**41**	**40.6**

As this table shows, there are no significant differences between cash clients and Title XX clients in terms of age, marital status and employment status, race, number of dependents, or dependence on other forms of public assistance. In other words, there is no discernible difference between cash clients and Title XX clients which would indicate that Title XX clients are unable to pay for their visits.

However, Medicaid clients appear significantly disadvantaged relative to cash or Title XX clients. Medicaid clients are significantly more likely to be minority, less educated, unmarried, unemployed, and on welfare, with more dependents.

Interestingly, Title XX funds represented 47% of PPHSET's revenues in 1985, while cash payments from clients represented 38%, and Medicaid funds added a mere 5%. Why would Title XX funds be almost ten times as important as Medicaid funds? And why would the demographics of Title XX and cash patients look almost identical?

The answers are to be found in the eligibility guidelines for the Title XX and Title XIX programs. The Title XIX (Medicaid) program is an entitlement program. Entitlement programs are designed to deliver basic needs to disadvantaged persons. Thus, the Medicaid program mandates an eligibility determination procedure that includes verifying and documenting the client's reported income. Medicaid eligibility is not determined at the clinic level, but at the government level, the state or county or city level. In order to receive Medicaid funding for her visit to Planned Parenthood, the client must bring her Medicaid card.

By contrast, the Title XX program mandates no eligibility requirements whatsoever. The federal government *recommends* that Title XX funds be used for poor people, but it imposes no such *requirement.*

Title XX eligibility is therefore determined at the clinic level, by clinic personnel, in accordance with state guidelines, if any. But the state guidelines are usually designed to ensure that the clinics can qualify virtually *anyone* for Title XX funding.

Consider, for example, this excerpt from a PPHSET memo to clinic directors, explaining how to qualify clients for Title XX:

Example 2: An 18-year-old patient states that she is a full-time college student. She is part-time employed with an average income of $50.00 per week. Her parents send her $150.00 per month for food. They also pay her tuition directly to the university. The student also uses her summer employment savings of $2000.00 to contribute to her monthly expenses. The student calculates that she uses about $150.00 a month to meet her other expenses. The patient is wearing three gold necklaces, two rings with multiple stones, one has rubies and diamonds, and the other has a black onyx stone with diamonds. She also has a Gucci purse and an obviously new pair of leather shoes. She states that her father is a banker and earns $35,000.00 a year and her mother is part-time employed with an income of $10,000.00 a year, the patient has two siblings.

Question: How is eligibility calculated and determined?

Answer: First and foremost, the patient is 18 years old, therefore she is a legal adult. Her parents and siblings are disregarded in determining eligibility. . . . This person would be Title XX eligible and assessed a co-pay of 20%.

Gucci shoes, diamond rings, money in the bank, college paid for, part-time job — hardly the picture of financial need or medical indigence! And yet, fully eligible for Title XX funding for her birth control visit. Struggling families who can't afford Gucci accessories and diamond rings, much less college educations, are being taxed to pay for wealthy girls to visit Planned Parenthood.

In Their Own Words

Another example from PPHSET demonstrates that non-Medicaid government funding of family planning is a waste of money because it is completely unnecessary. In the summer of 1986, PPHSET ran out of Title XX funds, which historically amount to about 50% of revenues. For several months, it was forced to go cold turkey, with its only federal funds being the relatively insignificant Medicaid funds (about 5% of total revenues). The clinics were forced to charge virtually all of their patients straight cash fees, even if they "qualified" for Title XX funding. No Title XX funds were available, period.

Of course, since the vast majority of their clients were indigents who could not afford to pay for their own birth control,

the clinics' revenues plunged as thousands of women were disen-
franchised from family planning services and forced to resort to
unplanned pregnancies or coat hanger abortions.

Well, no, actually, that's not what happened at all.

The minutes of the PPHSET Board of Directors meeting of
September 24, 1986, tell what really happened:

> Follow-up—If you recall at the Annual Meeting in May, I
> presented a pessimistic view of our financial condition going
> into the summer months. This was primarily due to our run-
> ning out of Title XX funding in Regions Eleven and Six.
>
> I am happy to report that the gloomy forecast did not come
> true, for a variety of reasons:
>
> • *Absent government funding, patients were willing to pay for their own
>   care.* [italics added]
>
> • The Brown and McAshan Foundations doubled their annual
>   contributions.
>
> • The Title XX billing was accelerated—meaning the money
>   was in our bank account, and not in the State of Texas!
>
> • The Lufkin and Tyler Clinics, which still had Title XX, con-
>   tinued to serve large numbers of patients.
>
> • Expenses were contained.

The Executive Director's Report at the January 21, 1987
Board Meeting reiterated that Title XX clients are willing and
able to pay for their own birth control visits:

> As I hope was mentioned in the Treasurer's Report, we finished
> 85/86 in the black. This success was due to a number of facts:
>
> • The Clinic staff successfully shifting patients to cash paying
>   status versus government funding. . . .

The Bigger Picture

Clearly, the purpose of Title XX funding is not what the
American taxpayer has been told—to provide family planning
services for indigents; the purpose is to provide a means for
Planned Parenthood clinics to generate increased business and
higher profits (would *you* pay your doctor for birth control pills if
you could get them "free" from Planned Parenthood?). The in-

evitable conclusion is that absent government funding, patients are both willing and able to pay for their own care because Title XX patients are not truly needy. Indeed, the national statistics corroborate this finding:[6]

CLIENTS OF FAMILY PLANNING PROGRAMS BY CHARACTERISTIC, BY YEAR

Year	White	Under 20 Years Old	Welfare Recipient
1969	40%	20%	N.A.
1973	N.A.	N.A.	17%
1983	70%	32%	13%

As family planning programs have expanded greatly under fifteen years of liberalized government funding, their client base has become significantly younger and, apparently, less poor: There are far fewer minorities and welfare clients. The main growth seems to have come primarily from white teen-aged girls, who, as we have seen, *automatically qualify* for government funding!

Chemical Racism

Title XX, nevertheless, allows Planned Parenthood clinics to target racial minorities for chemical sterilization and abortion services. As George Grant has effectively demonstrated in his book *Grand Illusions*,[7] Planned Parenthood has always been motivated by racist and eugenic philosophies, and has always targeted minorities, especially blacks and Hispanics, for sterilization (whether chemical or physical) and abortion.

Planned Parenthood's racist and eugenic origins have been well documented by feminists (such as the avowedly Marxist Linda Gordon in her book *Woman's Body, Woman's Right*) and by pro-life authors such as George Grant (*Grand Illusions*), Gary Bergel (*The Monstrosity of Planned Parenthood*), and Elisha Drogin (*Margaret Sanger, Father of Modern Society*). Gordon documents the following:

> The project was to hire three or four "colored ministers, prefer-
> ably with social-service backgrounds, and with engaging per-

---

6. Compiled from the Alan Guttmacher Institute, *Organized Family Planning Services in the United States, 1981-1983* (December, 1984), pp. 25-30.

7. George Grant, *Grand Illusions* (Nashville: Wolgemuth and Hyatt, 1988).

sonalities" to travel through the South and propagandize for birth control. "The most successful educational approach to the Negro is through a religious appeal." As Sanger wrote, in a private letter, "We do not want word to go out that we want to exterminate the Negro population and the minister is the man who can straighten out that idea if it ever occurs to any of their more rebellious members."[8]

Title XX funds represent the ideal means by which Planned Parenthood clinics can target minority populations for extinction, especially the Hispanic population, which has proved to be resistant to both contraception and abortion.

In 1985, PPHSET formed a Low Income Patients Task Force to develop a strategy for targeting poor people for family planning services. It also formed a Hispanic Task Force to determine how to reduce Hispanic fertility rates in the Houston area. Interestingly, these task forces found evidence that Hispanics' larger family sizes were due to Hispanics' desire for larger families; in other words, Hispanics were *planning* larger families.

The November 1986 issue of *Texas Medicine* contained an article that also supported the conclusion that high Hispanic fertility rates are not necessarily indicative of a lack of family planning, but to the contrary, result from Hispanics' desire for large families:

> Finally, to understand contraceptive trends, alternative explanations should be considered. Sabagh suggests that high fertility among Hispanic populations reflects a general desire by this cultural group for larger families. According to this hypothesis, a large proportion of pregnancies in this group, including adolescents, are planned. This reasoning suggests there are more children in this ethnic group primarily because the value of children is high. . . . In a relative sense, (at least for the state of Texas), the traditional recipient of indigent health care—the black population—is being quickly supplanted by a non-acculturated Hispanic population, especially the younger age groups. Whether this trend is largely because of the expanding Hispanic population, the general preference for larger families, or problems in contraceptive use, is unclear. This trend, if it continues, suggests that maternity services for the indigent in the 1990s will be dominated by cohorts of young, fertile, Hispanic

---

8. Linda Gordon, *Woman's Body, Woman's Right* (New York: Penguin Books, 1977), pp. 332-333.

women. In addition, immigration will continue to expand the childbearing pool with women who lack acculturation to the prevailing values of the larger society, especially as it relates to the value and worth of children and marriage.[9]

In other words, Hispanics have more children and larger families because they have not yet adopted Planned Parenthood's low regard for children and families. This conclusion is also supported by data from the U.S. Bureau of the Census:[10]

LIFETIME BIRTHS EXPECTED BY WIVES — 18-34 YEARS OLD — PERCENT DISTRIBUTION, 1985 DATA

Number of Births Expected	Race or Ethnicity		
	White	Black	Hispanic
None	6.4	3.6	4.1
One	12.6	14.1	9.1
Two	49.8	46.1	40.2
Three	22.2	21.8	26.0
Four or More	9.0	14.5	20.5

The larger family sizes that both blacks and Hispanics expect reflect their intentions and plans. We cannot attribute these expectations to a lack of access to, or utilization of, family planning services — because blacks and Hispanics are more frequent users of family planning services than whites:[11]

FAMILY PLANNING SERVICES — VISITS PER 1,000 WOMEN — 15-44 YEARS OLD, 1982 DATA

Source of Service	Race or Ethnicity		
	White	Black	Spanish Origin
Total	1,034	1,337	1,212
Private Medical Services	671	557	673
Clinics	323	756	524
Counselors	39	24	15

9. Peggy B. Smith, Ph.D. and Raymond Wait, M.D., "Adolescent Fertility and Childbearing Trends Among Hispanics in Texas," *Texas Medicine* 82 (November, 1986): 30-31.

10. United States Bureau of the Census, *Statistical Abstract of the Limited States: 1987* (107th edition). Washington, D.C., 1986, Table No. 97, p. 65.

11. Ibid., table no. 101, p. 67.

Thus, on a per capita basis Hispanics make 17% more family planning visits than whites, and blacks make 29% more visits than whites.

Nevertheless, organizations such as Planned Parenthood continue to target Hispanics on the perverse assumption that high fertility rates are bad *even if they are the result of deliberate, planned births*. This hypocritical assumption underlies the whole family planning mentality: Planned Parenthood values family planning only to the extent that family planning *reduces* family size; high birthrates are *ipso facto* considered to be conclusive proof of the need for more family planning.

It does not matter to Planned Parenthood that its family planning services may be unwanted; it intends to sell them. The minutes of the meeting of the Community Education Committee of PPHSET on November 24, 1986, underscore this attitude that minorities had better learn to like contraceptives and smaller families:

> David Smith provided a preliminary report on the current status and intentions of the LIPS [Low Income Patients] Task Force. . . . He suggested that the results will most likely confirm the earlier finding of the Hispanic Task Force study, which indicated that the Hispanic population in Southwest Houston is tremendously underserved by family planning services. Along with the recent immigrants from Latin America, teenagers still lack access *and motivation to utilize existing services*. [emphasis added]

Title XX plays a crucial role in targeting racial groups for fertility reduction. PPHSET's Low Income Patients Task Force Report (Draft) dated January 5, 1987 stated:

> Title XX is PPHSET's major source of funds. No income verification process is required to entitle a patient. Co-pay may be required and the system is flexible allowing for considerable discretion on the part of the interviewer. Undocumented patients can easily qualify under Title XX. All costs are reimbursed and if carefully managed a small profit margin can be maintained to help defray overhead costs.

The report went on to state that 90% of the patients seen at its Casa de Amigos clinic receive Title XX funding, and that in seven out of nine clinics, more than 50% of the clients receive Title XX funding. By being able to easily "qualify" minority clients for Title XX funding, Planned Parenthood is able to masquerade as a charitable benefactor to minority communities. Hispanics who cannot speak English probably cannot distinguish Title XX funding from Planned Parenthood's own philanthropy (which is virtually nonexistent); thus, Planned Parenthood is able to bill the taxpayer and take credit for the poor taxpayer's generosity.

It is interesting to note that while PPHSET admits that it earns a profit from servicing Title XX clients, the same Low Income Patients Task Force Report insisted that "abortions are not a moneymaker and costs have to be carefully watched."

The inescapable conclusion is that federal Title XX funds are being used to subsidize PPHSET's abortuary, something that Planned Parenthood insists does not happen.

Planned AntiParenthood

Title XX is by no means the only federal family planning program that is designed to qualify financially capable clients for government-paid family planning services. Both Title X and Title XX are intentionally designed to render parents completely irrelevant in their children's visits to Planned Parenthood. Neither program contains a parental consent or notification requirement, and teenagers qualify for government-paid birth control without regard to their parents' income.[12]

In fact, Planned Parenthood has ferociously fought off all federal attempts, and most state attempts, to require parental consent or parental notification, or to impose eligibility standards for Title X or XX funding based on the parents' income. Planned Parenthood successfully fought off a U.S. Department of Health and Human Services proposed regulation that would have re-

---

12. For example, the U.S. Department of Health and Human Services Title X regulations state, in part: " 'Low-income family' also includes members of families whose annual family income exceeds this amount, but who, as determined by the project director, are unable, for good reasons, to pay for family planning services. For example, unemancipated minors who wish to receive services on a confidential basis must be considered on the basis of their own resources." From 42 CFR 59.2, October 1, 1986 Edition. (Washington, D.C.: U.S. Government Printing Office).

quired clinics that receive Title X funds to charge fees for services based on parental income rather than the child's.

Obviously, virtually all unemancipated minors qualify as
"needy" based on their own income rather than that of their
parents!

Planned Parenthood vehemently denies that parents have an
interest in their children's sexual behavior that exceeds Planned
Parenthood's own interest. Planned Parenthood claims that it is
sincerely interested in reducing teen pregnancy and abortion
rates. Ironically, Planned Parenthood has been the single most
vigorous opponent of parental consent laws for birth control and
abortion, even though, or rather because, parental consent laws
have been shown to be an effective method to reduce the incidence of teen intercourse, pregnancy, abortion, and childbirth.
Across-the-board reductions in these undesired factors have
been achieved in states that have enacted parental consent legislation. According to the Alan Guttmacher Institute (founded by
Alan Guttmacher, a longtime leader of Planned Parenthood and
one of the main change agents responsible for the legalization of
abortion in America), mandatory parental involvement provisions result in a 24% to 85% reduction in teen caseloads at family planning clinics.[13]

It is extremely important to note that being able to provide
birth control devices to minors without parental knowledge or
consent or involvement in any way is fundamental to the mission *and survival* of Planned Parenthood. Planned Parenthood
simply cannot afford to have parents interfere with its secretive
provision of birth control and abortions to their children. To
allow such parental intrusion upon Planned Parenthood's fundamental right to profit from teen fornication would cripple Planned
Parenthood financially. Planned Parenthood is in reality not
concerned with reducing teen promiscuity; it is interested in
profiting from it.

An analysis of the clinic records from PPHSET demonstrates the crucial role of Title XX funding in facilitating teen
fornication: *97% of all unmarried minor girls who came to one of the
clinics for a birth control visit received Title XX funding, including 96%*

---

13. Alan Guttmacher Institute, *Issues in Brief* 4:3 (March, 1984).

of the girls who came to the clinic to get on birth control for the first time, and 93% of the girls who told Planned Parenthood not to send any mail to their home address. The provision of birth control to a minor daughter is strictly a matter between the daughter, the clinic, and the American taxpayer—parental input is neither required nor desired nor necessary. If Mom and Dad don't approve or won't pay, good ol' Uncle Sam will.

And so, the Title X and Title XX programs have been cleverly designed so that your teen-age daughter, yes, even your younger-than-teen-age daughter, can go to the nearest Planned Parenthood clinic and receive "free" government-funded birth control without your knowledge or consent.

No matter that providing birth control devices and chemicals to unmarried minors is considered to be a crime under some state statutes. No matter that providing birth control to your daughter may violate your religious convictions and undermine her moral training. No matter that providing birth control devices and chemicals to unmarried girls is to expose them to the likelihood of acquiring venereal diseases, such as herpes, gonorrhea, and the always fatal AIDS. No, none of these things matter to the federal government or to Planned Parenthood.

Rape and Incest: The Taxpayer as Victim

Qualifying young teens and financially healthy clients is not the only problem with Title XX funding for Planned Parenthood clinics. Despite the devious and dubious design of the Title XX eligibility qualification process, it would be a serious underestimation to assume that Planned Parenthood's interest in Title XX arises solely out of its ability to allow it to circumvent parental authority and to appear as a benefactor to certain targeted racial populations. Planned Parenthood has a pure profit motive in acquiring as many Title XX patients as possible.

Why? Because a Title XX patient is more profitable than a cash patient. *In all cases, Planned Parenthood bills more services and charges more fees when taxpayers are footing the bill than when the client pays cash.*[14] *To put it bluntly, Planned Parenthood is soaking the tax-*

---

14. The only exception would be when the purpose of visit was counseling—the average counseling visit cost twelve cents less for a government client.

payer. (Remember that these conclusions are based upon a statistical analysis of six thousand clinic visit records obtained from PPHSET, i.e., hard statistical data.)

COST OF A PREGNANCY TEST VISIT

Method of Payment	Average Total Cost	% of Total Clients
Cash, full-rate	$15.75	2%
Cash, reduced-rate[15]	$16.40	28%
Average cost, cash	**$16.36**	**30%**
Title XX	$57.93	67%
Medicaid	$47.18	3%
Average cost, govt.	**$57.51**	**70%**

The cost of a pregnancy test visit at Planned Parenthood is directly related to who's paying, the client or the taxpayer. *When the taxpayer pays, the pregnancy test visit is roughly three and a half times more expensive.*

To charge $57.93 for a pregnancy test visit is an *outrage*, no matter who's paying. To charge anything at all for a pregnancy test is shameful when you consider that there are thousands of crisis pregnancy centers (CPCs), private doctors, government health clinics, and abortion clinics that routinely perform free pregnancy testing.

Clearly, Planned Parenthood is charging cash clients much

---

15. The reader will note that the average amounts shown under "Cash, reduced-rate" sometimes slightly exceed the average amounts shown under "Cash, full-rate." This seeming incongruity arises because the amounts shown are totals for all services rendered during a visit. Thus, a reduced-rate patient may receive a higher total billing for a particular type of visit if she is billed for more services than a full-rate patient. Also, the discounts given to reduced-rate cash patients are generally rather small and apply to only some of the services and supplies. It should also be noted that the amounts shown under Title XX are understated by up to 20% because they do not include co-pay amounts charged directly to the patient. The amounts shown represent only those amounts charged directly to the government. The co-pay amount is similar to an insurance deductible for which the patient is directly responsible. If the co-pay amounts were included, the Title XX figures shown would be up to 25% higher. For instance, the average Title XX pregnancy test visit cost $66.46, of which $8.53 was paid in cash by the client and $57.93 was billed to the government.

less for their pregnancy tests primarily because that is all the market will bear: People won't pay much for a test that is performed free at most places or that can be done at home for ten dollars. It is not as if Planned Parenthood gives better results: You're either pregnant or you're not.

Further analysis of actual clinic records reveals that Planned Parenthood's excessive charges are not limited to pregnancy tests.

COST OF AN INITIAL BIRTH CONTROL VISIT

Method of Payment	Average Total Cost	% of Total Clients
Cash, full-rate	$63.01	1%
Cash, reduced-rate	$30.13	19%
Average cost, cash	**$32.13**	**20%**
Title XX	$77.55	78%
Medicaid	$63.81	2%
Average cost, govt.	**$77.20**	**80%**

COST OF AN ANNUAL BIRTH CONTROL VISIT

Method of Payment	Average Total Cost	% of Total Clients
Cash, full-rate	$73.14	3%
Cash, reduced-rate	$38.05	35%
Average cost, cash	**$40.60**	**38%**
Title XX	$85.83	61%
Medicaid	$69.58	1%
Average cost, govt.	**$85.20**	**62%**

COST OF A BIRTH CONTROL REPEAT VISIT

Method of Payment	Average Total Cost	% of Total Clients
Cash, full-rate	$22.14	1%
Cash, reduced-rate	$25.61	17%
Average cost, cash	**$25.37**	**18%**
Title XX	$35.94	80%
Medicaid	$25.16	2%
Average cost, govt.	**$35.77**	**82%**

COST OF A BIRTH CONTROL SUPPLY VISIT

Method of Payment	Average Total Cost	% of Total Clients
Cash, full-rate	$ 9.76	6%
Cash, reduced-rate	$10.34	68%
Average cost, cash	**$10.29**	**74%**
Title XX	$35.62	25%
Medicaid	$16.75	<1%
Average cost, govt.	**$35.47**	**26%**

Government clients are billed for more services at higher cost, regardless of the type of service rendered. Now, Planned Parenthood's counterargument for the higher billings for government-paid client visits is that Title XX patients are poorer and therefore have more health problems and less access to medical care. This would logically translate into more services and higher billings for each Title XX patient relative to cash patients.

Planned Parenthood's counterargument is false. It fails on three tests:

1. Logically, if Title XX patients were truly qualified based on need, we would expect the demographic profile of Title XX clients to closely resemble that of the Medicaid clients rather than that of the cash clients. However, as the table on page thirteen shows, such is not the case. The demographics of cash and Title XX patients are virtually identical, so we cannot conclude that Title XX patients require more services.

2. Planned Parenthood does not offer any routine nonsexually-oriented general medical care. Planned Parenthood is only concerned with sexual health, not general health. Thus, the general health of the patient is irrelevant in determining the scope of the services, for the available services are limited to birth control counseling and methods, pap smears and pelvic exams, abortions, and venereal disease diagnosis and treatment. Planned Parenthood is not treating coughs or heart disease or bad backs.

By analyzing the costs to just those clients who received an annual exam and physical, you still find that Title XX clients are billed at far higher rates ($73.83 versus $36.98 for cash clients). And if you look at just those clients who did not receive an annual exam and physical, you also find that Title XX clients are billed significantly higher rates ($25.46 versus $13.65 for cash clients). Clearly, routine health care services are not the explanation for why Title XX billings are so much higher.

3. Could it be that higher total billings for government-funded clients result from their use of services that are more expensive? Could it be that Title XX and Medicaid clients tend to go to Planned Parenthood for more expensive birth control services, while cash clients tend to go to Planned Parenthood for relatively less expensive venereal disease services?

Alas, such is not the case.

On average, Planned Parenthood charges from 140% to 350% more to service a government client, regardless of the type of service rendered.

The inescapable conclusion is that Planned Parenthood is systematically fleecing the taxpayer. Planned Parenthood consistently claims that it is saving the taxpayer money. If it honestly intended to do so, it wouldn't charge the government $57.93 for something the client could receive free elsewhere. In fact, if the pregnancy test client were to be tested at a crisis pregnancy center, not only would the government save the $57.93 for the pregnancy test, but it would likely save money on many other costs, too, since CPCs generally provide their services, including food, shelter, medical care, delivery, adoption, and postpartum care, at no cost.

Imagine the liberal media's indignation if Geraldo Rivera reported that crisis pregnancy centers charged 20% of their clients $16.36 cash for a pregnancy test, and billed the federal government at $57.93 for the other 80%!

Crisis Pregnancy Counseling: The Cash Connection

The PPHSET clinic records shed some light on the debate about the ethics of volunteer-staffed crisis pregnancy centers versus Planned Parenthood clinics/abortuaries. CPCs have been bashed by the media (and in Texas sued by the attorney general) because they have dared to present full information on prenatal development and on abortion. The death lobby and the liberal media are deeply offended because CPCs have dared to provide comprehensive pregnancy counseling — counseling that covers the moral, medical, emotional, and spiritual aspects of abortion and of motherhood—and because CPCs have dared to place a high value on an unborn child's life. (Abortionists place a high value on the baby's life, too—$150.00 to $2000.00, depending on gestation.)

CPCs have no profit motive, and they receive no government funds. Indeed, Department of Human Services regulations prohibit the funding of any project that does not refer for abortions.[16] CPCs exist solely to help new parents make plans for parenthood and to offer a comprehensive range of help for women who want to be the mothers of living children rather than dead children. Each woman seen by a CPC represents an unreimbursed financial expense for the organization.

Planned Parenthood, on the other hand, has a pure profit motive in administering pregnancy tests. Each pregnancy test client represents not only a potential $57.93 in revenues, but also a potential abortion customer.

Not only are taxpayers paying Planned Parenthood outlandish sums to perform pregnancy tests, we are also paying Planned Parenthood to counsel women *toward* abortion. Forty-nine percent of the women who came to PPHSET for a pregnancy test received "problem counseling." Problem counseling is *mandatory* for pregnant patients. Of course, this counseling is free for cash clients, but it costs $11.00 for Title XX clients. If the client receives a pregnancy test and is not pregnant, "initial education counseling" or "birth control method counseling" is mandatory. Of course, this counseling costs $7.00 each for Title XX clients but is provided free to most cash clients.

Not that you would have to *go* to the clinic to receive counseling. For Title XX patients, PPHSET will be glad to counsel you over the phone and then bill the government for problem counseling ($11.00).

And this counseling is enormously effective. *Out of the six thousand clinic visit records surveyed, including 724 records for clients who received pregnancy tests, there were only three referrals for adoption. Only one client who received problem counseling was referred for adoption. Abortions and abortion referrals outnumbered adoption referrals by more than fifty to one.*

---

16. Regulations in effect as of September 30, 1987.

Obviously, the whole situation is rigged to enrich Planned Parenthood at the expense of taxpayers and unborn children. It is ironic and terribly hypocritical that the organization that chants the mantra "every child a wanted child" with hypnotic consistency should be so biased against placing unborn children in homes where they are wanted.

A confidential survey conducted by Planned Parenthood Federation of America in 1986 found widespread confusion and ignorance at its affiliates concerning adoption. Thirty-five percent of Planned Parenthood affiliates surveyed opposed offering adoption services because adoption is inconsistent with the goals and practices of Planned Parenthood. These affiliates do not believe that Planned Parenthood should even offer adoption counseling — only referral. Only 20% of the affiliates expressed high enthusiasm for including adoption as part of Planned Parenthood's mission statement. (Adoption is *not* a part of Planned Parenthood's mission statement!)

Only 49% of the Planned Parenthood affiliates surveyed said that they could address the emotional issues that arise during the adoption process. Some of the affiliate comments were:

We offer brief counseling and usually don't offer much information about adoption, but counselors can respond to questions from clients. . . .

*   *   *

We do not know how to do private referrals [for adoptions] because we've never looked into the process.

*   *   *

Where yes has been checked, it refers to the minimal information given by our counselors when asked these specific questions by pregnant women.

In reply to the question, "Should adoption be part of Planned Parenthood's mission?", some typical responses included:

No. It would present an apparent and possibly actual conflict of interest. Difficult to finance. Very draining on staff time and overall effort.

*   *   *

At this point in time, I do not think adoption is an appropriate program for Planned Parenthood. We need to concentrate our resources on the areas clearly defined in our mission. I don't think we are doing these well enough to be looking at an adoption program.

*   *   *

Only as a referral. It might be very confusing to maintain a pro-choice stance when an agency also is invested in finding an infant to place.

*   *   *

I think we have to look very carefully at the issues involved. For our clients, we need to be sure that the information and services we provide are really in their best interest. A pregnant fifteen-year-old should not be seen as the "solution" to an infertile couple's problems. We need to be very careful not to cast women in the role of "baby producers" as if there were no effect on them if they place their infant for adoption. . . . I do think we need to provide better information about the issues around adoption — and we do need to be sure that the referral information we give out is accurate and useful.

*   *   *

We have historically presented adoption as an option in a most matter of fact way without presenting the whole picture. Of those patients who choose adoption, it only makes sense for us to be their mechanism to that end.

*   *   *

Planned Parenthood believes in choice, and all choices should be equally available and accessible. . . . The adoption agencies in (our) county have their own set of "additional" criteria, e.g., being a "born-again" Christian to be considered an adoptive parent. They decide who to reward with an infant and that leaves a lot of people out of the running. . . . Adoption, like abortion, has become a "political" issue. In (our) county it is viewed as "the" alternative regardless of the fact that few people are making this choice. I think that Planned Parenthood has a responsibility to see that people are not coerced into any choice. . . . "If" Title X dollars are going to be allowed to be used for adoption, I think we should position ourselves to use them.

*   *   *

I strongly believe that adoption is a valid method of achieving parenthood and therefore believe it should be part of our mission. I also believe that we have not put enough research, energy, and resources in this option.

It is not hard to see why only a fraction of 1 percent of Planned Parenthood's clients are being referred for adoption. It is sickening to see taxpayers forced to pay for pro-abortion, antiadoption "problem counseling" while at the same time CPCs are denied federal funding because they refuse to refer for abortions. For Planned Parenthood, pregnancy testing, problem counseling, and abortion are one slick package all wrapped up in Title XX funding.

If Saving Taxpayers Money Is the Intention, Why Is Spending Taxpayers' Money the Goal?

Considering that Medicaid and Title XX clients are so profitable, it is not surprising to find that Planned Parenthood actively recruits both types of clients. For instance, a draft of the minutes of the October 31, 1986, PPHSET clinic directors' meeting included the following goals:

Sally Miller—Brazos Clinic
  • Increase Title XX patients

Verneal Smith—Smith Clinic
  • Patient Statistics—Low, we had increase this week
    Working hard to increase flow of patients
  • Moving toward spending Title XX dollars

Diane Wheeler—Angelina County Clinic
  • Patient Status—550 patients last month
    Averaging thirty patients a day
  • Working on increasing Medicaid patients

Tina Gano — Casa Amigos Clinic
- Goal to increase patient statistics

II. Fiscal update

David Goodrich — Director of Finance briefly went over many financial aspects which include:
- Financial Statement Sheet — No Title XX — no money, with Title XX — make money Projected Revenue — Brings Cash in — (let's try to make our goal every month)

In fact, the clinic distributes flyers that promise a "ten percent discount off next exam or free gift for Medicaid patients." These flyers are also printed in Spanish and have been sent to local housing projects for distribution.

Medicaid clients are valuable because Medicaid is an entitlement program, meaning that money is always available to fund Medicaid services.[17] By contrast, Title XX funds are block grant funds that are limited to the annual federal and state allocations; Title XX funds sometimes run out before the end of the fiscal year.

It should come as no surprise that Planned Parenthood is also interested in increasing its abortion volume. Planned Parenthood is always insisting that it wants to reduce abortion, but this is just public posturing. PPHSET worked with Problem Pregnancy, Inc., to generate Texas abortion clients for California and New York abortionists starting in 1972.[18] And then after *Roe v. Wade*, PPHSET opened Houston's first legal abortuary. Houston's Planned Parenthood budgets abortions as a revenue line item, and it tracks abortion volume on a monthly "Performance Checklist." An internal memo dated April 7, 1986, from PPHSET's Deputy Executive Director discussed a proposal to increase the

---

17. Planned Parenthood successfully lobbied Congress in 1986 and 1987 to revise the Medicaid program to ensure that Planned Parenthood did not lose some of its clients to HMOs or family practitioners. Congress passed provisions that mandated that Medicaid recipients who enrolled in HMOs or other provider plans, voluntarily or involuntarily, could nevertheless obtain family planning services from an outside provider. These changes did a lot more to protect Planned Parenthood from competition than to ensure that poor women continue to receive family planning prescriptions.

18. Planned Parenthood of Houston and Southeast Texas, "Proud of Our Past, Planning the Future, 50 Years of Planned Parenthood," (Houston: 1986).

clinic's abortion business by making abortion an all-in-one-visit process rather than a two-visit process:

> The immediate change I would like to discuss is a revision in our patient flow for clients desiring an abortion. . . . This change will probably increase patient volume and therefore result in increased revenue. Resistance may come from both clinic and medical staff. . . .

Although PPHSET charges $150.00 *cash only* for an abortion up to twelve weeks, it does of course provide a $25.00 discount for Medicaid patients. At $47.18 average cost for a Medicaid client's pregnancy test, the discount seems appropriate.

Summary

In its misguided attempt to reduce dependency on government welfare programs, the government has created a new dependent class: Planned Parenthood clinics. These clinics have a vested interest in promoting and encouraging teen fornication; profiting from teen fornication and its attendant side effects is Planned Parenthood's business. Planned Parenthood has become the enemy of the unborn, of the taxpayer, of blacks and Hispanics, and most ironic of all, of parents. Planned Parenthood's insatiable desire for more and more tax dollars has led it to oppose chastity programs and parental consent laws, because reducing teen fornication spells disaster for Planned Parenthood.

The government's grand experiment in subsidizing the chemical and surgical sterilization of the poor through government support of Planned Parenthood (and other family planning/abortion programs) has been a miserable failure. The main recipients of government subsidy are financially capable, white, teen-age girls who receive no other form of welfare.

Planned Parenthood has used its profits from government programs to target racial minorities for sterilization (permanent or chemical), to subsidize its abortuaries, to lobby elected officials, to finance lawsuits against pro-lifers and against pro-life legislation, and to criticize crisis pregnancy centers while it provides biased, pro-abortion, antiadoption pregnancy counseling.

Planned Parenthood clinics are using these government funding programs to circumvent and nullify just parental concerns, and to cheat taxpayers by systematically and deliberately pumping up the billings for government-funded clients. Planned Parenthood's incestuous relationship with the federal government has led to a gang rape of the taxpayer by Planned Parenthood clinics.

In the interest of fiscal sanity, family sanctity, and racial equality, it's time to defund Planned Parenthood.

CHALKBOARD EVAN-GELISTS: SELLING SEX IN THE CLASSROOM

Planned Parenthood believes deeply, passionately in sex education. In recent years, Planned Parenthood has come to promote a more insidious kind of sex education than mere biological sex education. This new brand of sex education allegedly seeks to help students develop decision-making skills and coping skills, and to explore their own personal feelings and values and options in regard to the question of fornication.

I say fornication, because the explicit focus of the new sex-ed programs is on sex outside of heterosexual, monogamous marriage. The context of the courses is that sex is a whole-life, birth-to-death concept and that therefore all human beings can be legitimately "sexually active" at any stage in their lives, regardless of marital status.

In these courses, sex is not taught as something that was designed primarily for procreation and secondarily for enjoyment and fulfillment, and these between a husband and a wife in an "until-death-do-us-part" marriage. Rather, sex is taught as a normal range of recreational/pleasurable acts between a teenager and his or her *partner*. What is right is whatever's right *for you*, regardless of the two-thousand-year-old teachings of the Church, or state laws limiting sexual contact between unmarried minors or homosexuals, or the accumulated moral teachings of thousands of years of western civilization.

These new sex-ed courses often come disguised under a variety of headings, such as *Family Life Education*.

Oftentimes, these courses are broken into sections that are integrated into a broad spectrum of unrelated courses including English, social studies, world history, and the like. Very often, these courses are taught without textbooks, using only materials that cannot be taken home for parental review.

According to Planned Parenthood Federation of America (PPFA), a comprehensive sex education course contains at least four of the following topics: biological facts about reproduction, talk about coping with your sexual development, information about different kinds of birth control, information about preventing sexual abuse, facts about abortion, facts about where to get contraceptives.[1] *Notice that PPFA considers sex-ed courses that completely ignore venereal diseases, sexual morality, religion, and AIDS to be comprehensive.*

Planned Parenthood's definition of a comprehensive sex-ed course reveals its fatally flawed belief in the primary importance of *birth control*. To Planned Parenthood, fornication is not a sin, but being pregnant *is*. Thus, Planned Parenthood never seeks to reduce teen promiscuity; rather it always seeks to reduce teen birthrates through abortion and other birth control methods. Indeed, Planned Parenthood often treats teen sex as therapeutic, enriching, fulfilling, rewarding, fun, almost as a positive good. To Planned Parenthood, even pregnancy is not as bad as one might suppose: The real threat is childbirth.

Thus, Planned Parenthood conveys the message that while teen sex is almost a sinless, sacred act, teen childbirth is a grave moral wrong. This perverted doctrine is exactly backwards: Teen fornication is a sin, but it is never a sin to be pregnant or to give birth, regardless of one's marital status. It's not that Planned Parenthood's teaching is secular or amoral: It is religiously immoral.

Isn't it really a little over-hyping the matter to say that Planned Parenthood's sexual teachings are religious? Not if you believe Planned Parenthood.

For instance, in 1983 PPFA published a magazine entitled *Religion: A Key Foundation for Family Life Education.* This magazine

---

1. Humphrey Taylor, Michael Kagay, Ph.D., and Stuart Leichenko, *American Teens Speak: Sex, Myths, TV, and Birth Control* (New York: Louis Harris and Associates, Inc., 1986), p. 47.

included articles on the fundamental interrelation between religion, beliefs, values, and sexual behavior. Of course, those values are always "loving" and "caring" and "growing" and "sharing" and "responding" and "nurturing," to the exclusion of "obedience" or "holiness" or "righteousness" or "faithfulness" or "godliness."

While many professing Christians hesitate to promote their religious beliefs regarding sex, Planned Parenthood does not. PPHSET sponsored a seminar for clergymen to teach churches how to instruct their youth groups in "sexuality." This seminar was entitled, "Be Fruitful and Multiply"[2] and was to be taught by Meryl Cohen. For this seminar, Susan Nenney, the associate director of communications at the abortuary, prepared a memo that summarized the theology of Planned Parenthood and its applicability to churches. This memo read in part:

> While our humanity is welcomed as a gift from God, we often hesitate to accept with equal joy our sexuality as a natural part of that gift. But religion and sexuality are interrelated. Religion has much to say to us about our sexual responsibility, and the decisions we make about sexuality reflect our religious beliefs.
> . . . In and through expression of sexuality we learn to trust one another, and trust is the basis of faith.

(Lest any reader believe that Planned Parenthood is asserting Scriptural views of sexuality here, we should note that a few months after she wrote this memo, Susan Nenney stated on a Houston radio talk show that Planned Parenthood does not view premarital sex, or any other kind of sex, as a sin. She asserted that Planned Parenthood does not believe in the concept of sin.)

Interestingly, the Meryl Cohen who was to conduct the seminar asserting the interrelatedness of sex and religion was the same Meryl Cohen who helped develop the Houston Independent School District's *Family Life Education* course, an immoral, no-textbook "comprehensive" sex education course that contained such gems of wisdom as the "fact" that abstinence is not an abso-

---

2. An ironic and cynical title for a seminar sponsored by an organization which aborts 100,000 children per year in America alone. See Planned Parenthood Federation of America, *1987 Planned Parenthood Service Report*, New York, 1987.

lute safeguard against pregnancy or venereal disease.[3] (I doubt they were extrapolating data obtained from Nazareth two thousand years ago.) This course also promotes the outright lie that *anyone* can get venereal disease. But *anyone* cannot get venereal disease. To get venereal disease, you have to have sexual contact with an infected person; people who practice chastity or faithful monogamous marriage cannot catch venereal disease.

Obviously, Planned Parenthood is merely doing its standard job of misinforming impressionable young minds to build in certain biases in favor of promiscuity. Planned Parenthood routinely classifies chastity or abstinence as a method of contraception equivalent to taking the Pill or using condoms or diaphragms. But since sex, especially premarital sex, is so much *fun*, Planned Parenthood treats the Pill and condoms and IUDs and diaphragms and sponges as the only serious and practical birth control methods, while it offers chastity no real support other than to mention it in passing as a theoretically effective method of birth control.

Planned Parenthood's sex education contains many other glaring examples of *disinformation*. For instance, Planned Parenthood has redefined abstinence to mean not having vaginal intercourse rather than abstaining from all sexual activity. To Planned Parenthood, ejaculating outside a girl's vagina or ejaculating into her mouth is abstinence.

This Planned Parenthood-designed HISD sexual how-to course is being taught to sixth graders in coeducational classes. The course includes the information that "it's alright to say no." But it is not "alright" to say no; saying no to fornication and its curses is

---

3. Unfortunately, the course's misinformation on venereal disease was not limited to disparaging the efficacy of abstinence. Here are the curriculum's five "ways to prevent the spread of AIDS": "1. Maintain good personal health. Get plenty of rest, eat a nutritious diet, and exercise regularly. 2. Reduce emotional stress. Learn positive ways to deal with problems. Stress decreases the body's ability to resist disease. 3. Avoid the abuse of all drugs. Do not share intravenous needles. 4. Choose to say no to having sex. Such practices as anal intercourse and oral-genital contacts are known to increase the risk of transmitting the AIDS virus. Any practices that may cause injury to the vaginal or anal tissues should be avoided. 5. Follow safe habits of cleanliness at all times." Apparently, the transmission of AIDS is related to whether you wash behind your ears and eat your vegetables.

not one acceptable option, but the *only* acceptable option. And it is totally unacceptable to say yes to fornication and sodomy.

Planned Parenthood also does a masterful job of redefining *responsibility*. Parents in the HISD were repeatedly assured that the course would teach sexual responsibility. But never was abstinence taught as responsible, nor was fornication ever taught as irresponsible. All-in-all, responsibility turned out to mean using contraception and avoiding childbirth by getting an abortion.

Although the course was designed to highlight the normally burdensome consequences of unmarried teen childbirth, Planned Parenthood as usual refused to draw the conclusion that unmarried teens should therefore not engage in intercourse. No, Planned Parenthood's implication was that teens should use contraception and abortion to avoid childbirth.

When the HISD school board was confronted with the moral bankruptcy of the program, it responded untruthfully by insisting that the program was being revised to stress abstinence. In addition, one school board member, an elderly woman named Elizabeth Spates, demanded that those who were opposed to the program submit a better way to solve the district's pregnancy crisis. She related that two nine-year-old girls had attended an HISD school for pregnant mothers the previous year, and that was the reason this program was so greatly needed.

No one bothered to explain to Ms. Spates that teaching sixth graders how to have sex could not possibly prevent third graders from getting pregnant. However, Ms. Spates did go on to say that she realized that education alone would not work, *which is why she supported mandatory licensing of parents before they could have children*.

But worse than the factual inaccuracies and theological heresies of the program are the flawed misconceptions and myths upon which it is based. Planned Parenthood likes to paint itself as the picture of sexual enlightenment, bringing reason and knowledge to legions of sexual idiots.

The facts, however, say otherwise.

In 1986, Planned Parenthood contracted Louis Harris and Associates to conduct a nationwide poll of teen sex attitudes, beliefs, and behavior. The results of this poll were released in late 1986 in a booklet entitled *American Teens Speak: Sex, Myths,*

TV, and Birth Control.[4] This amazing poll revealed that it is Planned Parenthood, not teen-agers, that clings to dangerous sexual myths. Virtually every major finding of this poll directly contradicts the conventional wisdom about teens and sex education. This poll destroys the practical, statistical, and philosophical basis on which Planned Parenthood designs and promotes its programs.

Some of the major myths that were exploded were:

Myth #1. Everybody's doing it. Everybody is not doing it. Only 28% of all teens have ever had sexual intercourse (this figure was not adjusted by the bragging factor). Only 4% of twelve-year-olds have ever had intercourse. More than three-fourths of American teen-age girls report that they are virgins and practice chastity, and more than two-thirds of teen-age boys report the same thing.[5]

Myth #2. Minorities fornicate more than whites. The study did not address the issue of how often nonvirgins fornicate. It did, however, address the percentages of virgins among blacks, whites, and Hispanics. The study showed no significant difference in rates of first-time intercourse between whites and Hispanics, but it did show that blacks are significantly less likely to remain virgins at any given age. Overall, the percentage of black virgins was twenty-three percentage points less than for whites. However, race alone is insufficient to account for differences in rates of first-time intercourse, because the study found significant differences based on frequency of attendance at religious services, grade point averages, economic status, geographic location, parents' education, college plans, and employment status.[6]

Only a racist could conclude that blacks have higher rates of first-time intercourse due to some genetic or biological difference. Obviously, the higher rate of black first-time intercourse

---

4. *American Teens Speak: Sex, Myths, TV, and Birth Control*, subtitled "The Planned Parenthood Poll." Conducted for the Planned Parenthood Federation of America; fieldwork performed September-October 1986. The full text of this poll is available from Louis Harris and Associates, Inc., 630 Fifth Avenue, New York, New York 10111.

5. *American Teens Speak*, p. 15.

6. Ibid., p. 16.

results from higher relative distributions of blacks in other socio-
logical classifications such as low income, parents not college
graduates, no plans to attend college, single parent households,
and the like. The causes of black teen promiscuity are greater
social and peer pressure to have sex, impaired family structures,
and the failure of our public schools to inculcate high achievement standards and high long-term goals. The most effective
way to reduce black teen promiscuity is to do a better job of educating and motivating students rather than wasting precious
educational time discussing how to do something they shouldn't
be doing.

Myth #3. Teen-agers have sex because it's natural. Reasons such as
peer pressure or "everyone's doing it" were cited by three times
more teen-agers than sexual feelings or desires as reasons that
teen-agers engage in sexual intercourse. In fact, 90% of teens
who have had sexual intercourse cited some variant of peer pressure or social pressure as a reason why teens engage in sex, while
only 10% cited "love," 12% cited sexual gratification, and 20%
cited curiosity.[7] Clearly, most teen-agers have sex because Planned
Parenthood and TV and school sexual how-to courses foster a
false panic that everyone's doing it.

Myth #4. Teen-agers are not interested in delaying sex. Seventy-
nine percent of all teens believe that teen-agers start having sex too
soon. Three out of four teen-agers believe that teen-agers should
wait until they are adults before engaging in sexual intercourse.[8]

Myth #5. Teen-agers want easier access to birth control. Seven out
of eight teenagers do not want a contraceptive-dispensing clinic
in their schools. Sixty percent do not even want clinics that dispense contraceptives located anywhere close to their schools.

---

7. Ibid., p. 24. Responses were recategorized by this author to correct
some misattributions in the survey. For instance, Planned Parenthood wrongly
categorized "makes you feel cool" under "Sexual Feelings/Desires" rather than
under the correct category of "Social Pressure." Similarly, it miscategorized
"want to feel grown up" under the category of "Curiosity" rather than under
"Social Pressure."

8. Ibid., p. 18.

Even six out of seven teen-agers who fornicate do not want a contraceptive-dispensing clinic in their schools.[9]

Myth #6. Teen sex is subject to prior education and planning, or most teens would use birth control if they knew how to get it and could get it easily. Unfortunately, teen fornication is incredibly resistant to contraception. First, the largest percentage (39%) of teens said that teens do not use birth control *simply because they prefer not to do so.*[10] In addition, two-thirds of all teens who have had intercourse say that their first act of intercourse was unexpected, that it "just happened."[11] Teen fornicators who do not use birth control cited the spontaneous nature of their sexual adventures more than two to one over any other reason for not using birth control. *In addition, "prefer not to use" or "no time to use" were cited by fornicators 428% more often than "lack of knowledge or access" as reasons for not using birth control.* Only 14% of sexually active teens who do not use birth control cited "lack of knowledge or access" as the main reason for failure to use protection. According to the survey, teenage fornicators say that the spontaneous, unanticipated nature of their sexual adventures is the main reason they do not use birth control.[12] Bottom line, teen-agers are engaging in spontaneous sex, and a huge proportion simply prefer not to use birth control or to use it only when convenient.

The issue is not sexual *knowledge*; it's sexual *behavior*.

Myth #7. Most teens believe a lot of stupid myths about sex that only sex education courses can correct. Both premises are false. Planned Parenthood's survey revealed a remarkably small level of mythical misinformation among teens. Planned Parenthood concludes that "a majority of teenagers do give the right answers when confronted with some of the most dangerous myths that circulate in teenage society."[13]

Actually, the greatest area of sexual ignorance seems to lie in Planned Parenthood. Planned Parenthood believes in *all* of the

---

9. Ibid., p. 71.
10. Ibid., p. 27.
11. Ibid., p. 26.
12. Ibid., p. 28.
13. Ibid., p. 29.

myths debunked in this chapter, even when its own research dis-proves them. And Planned Parenthood continues to spew a flood of sexual misinformation and myths to mislead American teens. For instance, the survey said that it is "usually true" that "a girl cannot become pregnant if she has intercourse during her menstrual periods."[14]

But Planned Parenthood is wrong. Any woman could have a biological misfunction that would enable her to be impregnated during menstruation, although such events are rare. Thus, the correct answer is neither "usually true" nor "usually false," the two options given by Planned Parenthood. The question as stated is a matter of fact ("cannot"), not a matter of probability ("usually will not"). The choice of the responses renders the question totally worthless. Planned Parenthood also asked teens whether it is "usually true" or "usually false" that "it is possible for a girl to become pregnant even though her male partner's penis did not actually enter her vagina." The question "is it *possible?*" is either *true* or *false*, but cannot be *usually true* or *usually false*. The question asked is "is it *possible?*" not "is it *likely?*" Planned Parent-hood claims that the correct answer is "usually true." Thus, the appalling conclusion is that Planned Parenthood is informing teen-agers that a girl who has intercourse during her menstrual period is unlikely to get pregnant, whereas a girl who does not have sexual intercourse is likely to become pregnant. What total hogwash! This is sex education?

The Houston Independent School District *Family Life Educa-tion* curriculum co-authored by Meryl Cohen of PPHSET is full of misleading statements designed to convey similar impres-sions, such as that condoms are almost totally effective but absti-nence does not provide any guarantees that you will not get pregnant or catch a sexually transmitted disease. Apparently, Planned Parenthood believes that AIDS is never spread by casual contact, but pregnancy often is.

Myth #8. Sex education results in sexually knowledgeable teens. Although sex education does result in an increase in some teens' sexual knowledge, the majority of teens who have had a compre-

---

14. Ibid., p. 32.

hensive sex education course still fail to exhibit what Planned
Parenthood considers a high level of sexual knowledge.[15] But
much of the increase in sexual knowledge for teens who have
had comprehensive sex-ed courses can be explained by the far
higher rates of teen promiscuity among those students.[16] *Thus,
we can say that Planned Parenthood-style "comprehensive" sex education
courses increase teens' sexual knowledge by increasing teen sexual activity.*

Myth #9. Sex education can change teen sexual attitudes and behaviors so that sexually active teens will use birth control. The survey reveals that only 40% of sexually active students who have taken a
comprehensive sex-ed course regularly use contraception. Thus,
60% of all students who have taken a comprehensive sex-ed
course and who are sexually active do not consistently practice
contraception. The comparable regular-use figures are 30% for
students who have had a noncomprehensive sex-ed course and
25% for students who have had no sex education course.[17] Obviously, neither biological sex education nor comprehensive sex
education courses offer any hope of stemming the fallout from
teen fornication. At best, six out of ten sexually active teens will
still remain at very high risk for pregnancy, and at least eight out
of ten will remain at very high risk for AIDS, incurable herpes,
gonorrhea, syphilis, chlamydia, and other venereal diseases. It
might be argued, however, that at least comprehensive sex education makes *some* improvement in the percentage of teens practicing effective contraception. However, comprehensive sex-ed
courses increase the number of sexually active teens by an even
greater amount, so that the net effect of a comprehensive sex
education course is to increase the number of sexually active
teens as well as the number of sexually active teens who do not
regularly use contraception.[18]

---

15. Ibid., p. 52.

16. Ibid., pp. 33, 53, 55, and 59. Of teens who have had sexual intercourse,
48% scored high on the Planned Parenthood's sexual knowledge level quiz,
while only 13% scored low. Corresponding rates for virgins were 28% who
scored high and 28% who scored low.

17. Ibid., p. 59.

18. Ibid., pp. 53, 59; see also footnote 21 in this chapter, as well as Myth 10.

Myth #10. Contraceptive-oriented sex education courses do not encourage teen fornication; rather, they are effective in decreasing teen promiscuity and teen pregnancies. Wrong again. While *biological* sex-ed courses do not increase teen promiscuity, *contraceptive-oriented sex-ed courses are correlated with an astounding 50% higher rate of teen promiscuity!*[19] Only 32% of students who have had no sex education have engaged in sexual intercourse, compared to 46% of students who have had a "comprehensive" sex education course. (Students who took a biological or noncomprehensive sex-ed course had about the same rate of intercourse as teens who had no sex-ed — 30%).[20]

In addition, comprehensive sex education courses are correlated with a 31% increase in both the rate and the absolute number of teens engaging in sexual intercourse without regular contraception.[21]

Even the Alan Guttmacher Institute has published studies that have concluded that sex education does not reduce teen promiscuity or teen pregnancy. For instance, the July/August 1986 issue of *Family Planning Perspectives* contained a study entitled "The Effects of Sex Education on Adolescent Behavior." This study concluded that sex education is a failure:

> It is widely believed that providing teenagers with information about pregnancy and birth control is crucial if the incidence of adolescent pregnancy is to be reduced, and that formal sex education programs are an appropriate and important vehicle for providing information. . . . Between 57 percent and 65 percent of teenagers receive formal contraceptive instruction before initiating coitus. However, our analyses fail to show any consistent relationship between exposure to contraceptive edu-

---

19. Calculated from *American Teens Speak*, p. 53.
20. Ibid.
21. Ibid., pp. 53, 59. Method of calculation: Of 1000 students who have had a biological, noncomprehensive sex-ed course, 30% will have had sexual intercourse and 70% of those will not practice regular contraception. Thus, the number of sexually active students who do not use regular contraception is $1000 \times (70\%) \times (30\%) = 210$. Of 1000 students who have taken a comprehensive sex-ed course, 46% will have had sexual intercourse :and 60% of those will not practice effective contraception. Thus the number of sexually active students who do not use effective contraception is $1000 \times (46\%) \times (60\%) = 276$, or 31% more than the noncomprehensive sex-ed group.

cation and subsequent initiation of intercourse. . . . The final
result to emerge from the analysis is that neither pregnancy
education nor contraceptive education exerts any significant
effect on the risk of premarital pregnancy among sexually active teenagers — a finding that calls into question the argument
that formal sex education is an effective tool for reducing
adolescent pregnancy.[22]

Other studies have found that sex education courses actually
increase the likelihood of starting intercourse for fifteen- and
sixteen-year-olds, and that any increases in contraceptive usage
rates are offset by increases in the number of teens having sex:

> Adolescent women who have previously taken a sex education
> course are somewhat more likely than those who have not to in-
> itiate sexual activity at ages 15 and 16. . . . Among the strong-
> est determinants of first coitus at those ages are infrequent
> church attendance, parental education of fewer than 12 years
> and black race. Older sexually active girls who have previously
> had a course are significantly more likely to use an effective
> contraceptive method (73 percent) than are those who have
> never taken a course (64 percent). This relationship may offset
> any effect that a sex education course may have in raising the
> likelihood of early first coitus, since no significant association
> can be found between taking a sex education course and subse-
> quently becoming premaritally pregnant before age 20.[23]

22. Alan Guttmacher Institute, "The Effects of Sex Education on Adolescent Behavior," Family Planning Perspectives, 18:4 (July/August, 1986), pp.
162, 169.

23. Alan Guttmacher Institute, William Marsiglio and Frank L. Mott,
"The Impact of Sex Education on Sexual Activity, Contraceptive Use and
Premarital Pregnancy Among American Teenagers," Family Planning Perspectives, 18:4 (New York: Alan Guttmacher Institute, July/August, 1986). It
should be noted that this study found that while sex education courses raised
the rates of first-time sexual intercourse among nonwhites by 20%, the
courses had no significant effect on their contraceptive usage; the inescapable
conclusion is that sex education courses significantly exacerbate the teen pregnancy problem among nonwhites. This study also found that "[t]he strongest
determinants of first intercourse at age fifteen are church attendance no more
than several times a year, parental education of fewer than 12 years, and black
race," which is probably another way of saying "lack of moral guidance, lack of
positive reasons for delaying intercourse and pregnancy, and an abundance of
peer pressure."

The most significant effect of a comprehensive sex-ed course, then, is to increase teen fornication rates by about 50%, and all sex-related problems (pregnancy, venereal disease, abortion, emotional distress, etc.) by about 31% to 50%.[24]

Myth #11. Parents don't talk to their children about sex. Parents were cited most often by students as their greatest source of information about how pregnancy is caused, and about contraception and birth control.[25] In addition, more than two-thirds of all teen-agers report that they have discussed sex with their parents, including 64% of twelve- and thirteen-year-olds.[26] By contrast, *parents were cited twenty-one times more often than Planned Parenthood as actual sources of information about how pregnancy is caused.*[27] Clearly, most parents talk to their children about sex, and most do it very early, long before their children are likely to be confronted with the issue on a practical level.

Myth #12. Having parents talk to their children about birth control reduces the rate of teen promiscuity and pregnancy. Thirty-two percent of teens whose parents did not talk to them about sex or birth control have had sex. Twenty-five percent of those teens whose parents spoke with them about sex *but not birth control* have engaged in sexual intercourse. Thus the children of parents who talked with them about sex *but not birth control* are somewhat less likely to be sexually active. However, 47% of teens whose parents have discussed both sex *and* birth control with them have had premarital sex.[28] Thus, we conclude that it is important that parents not discuss birth control with their children unless they want them to become sexually active.

---

24. Assuming, as does *American Teens Speak*, that the correlation between higher promiscuity and comprehensive sex-ed courses is due to a causal relationship rather than a coincidence. This assumption is reasonable, since sex education must be assumed to influence sexual behavior or there would be no justification for sex education courses. It could be argued that comprehensive sex-ed courses have been instituted primarily in high-promiscuity school districts. If such were the case, there does not seem to be any evidence that they are reducing promiscuity or unintended pregnancies.

25. *American Teens Speak*, p. 41.

26. Ibid., p. 43.

27. Ibid., p. 41.

28. Ibid., p. 45.

Myth #13. Scaring kids into chastity won't work. Most students say that three things would be effective in persuading teen-agers to remain chaste: (1) Telling them to worry more about catching diseases like AIDS and herpes (65%), (2) Telling them how a pregnancy could ruin their lives (62%), and (3) Telling them to worry more about what their parents would say or do to them if they found out (50%).[29] Clearly, Planned Parenthood's sex-ed courses that downplay the risks of venereal disease and portray abortion as a readily available option only aggravate the problem. And, just as clearly, Planned Parenthood's refusal to obtain parental permission before furnishing birth control information, devices, and drugs only adds to teen promiscuity.

Myth #14. Moral or religious approaches to teen promiscuity cannot work. Surprise! Teens who attend religious services frequently are less than half as likely to engage in fornication than teens who seldom or never attend religious services. Indeed, while attending so-called comprehensive sex-ed courses is correlated with 50% higher teen promiscuity rates, attending religious services frequently is correlated with one-third lower teen promiscuity rates.[30] Clearly, an approach to sex education that reinforces chastity, rules out premarital sex as immoral, and emphasizes the devastating consequences of teen promiscuity (AIDS, other venereal diseases, pregnancy) could result in a real lessening of teen promiscuity rates. This approach would not only agree with the real finding of Planned Parenthood's teen sex survey as to *what works*, but would also greatly reduce the peer pressure/social pressure that is the overwhelming reason cited by teens as the main cause of teen fornication.

Facing Reality

Students are crying out for their schools to promote healthy atmospheres that reinforce and encourage their predominantly chaste, virginal lifestyles. The primary cause of student fornication is peer pressure, and students clearly do not want the added peer pressure of school-based sex clinics or coed sex education

29. Ibid., p. 60.
30. Ibid., p. 16. This inverse correlation between religiosity and promiscuity is an almost universally documented aspect of teen sexuality.

classes. Students are looking for excuses to say no, not mechanical or chemical sexual aids to make fornication "safer." Virginity and abstinence are normative in teen-agers; fornication and promiscuity remain aberrational behaviors.

When either parents or schools teach students about birth control methods, abortion, how to obtain contraceptives, and the like, they significantly aggravate the problem of teen promiscuity. Indeed, the entire premise of Planned Parenthood's sex education, that teen promiscuity and pregnancy is the result of teens' lack of sexual information and lack of access to birth control chemicals and devices, is *totally* wrong; in fact, exactly backwards. The more teens are told about birth control and how to get it, the more likely they are to be sexually active *but still not use birth control*. Teen promiscuity does not stem from a lack of sexual knowledge; sexual information or birth control information are ineffective, indeed, *counterproductive*, weapons in the war on teen promiscuity and teen pregnancy.

As the main proponent of contraceptive-oriented sex-ed courses, Planned Parenthood is clearly the major source of the myths about sex. Planned Parenthood's "comprehensive" sex education courses are not the cure, they are the disease; they are not the solution to the problem, *they are the problem*.

Planned Parenthood has done the pro-family movement a tremendous service by publishing this teen sex poll. The results flatly contradict every major premise of sex education. Unfortunately, Planned Parenthood totally ignored the major findings of the poll and drew conclusions that were totally opposed to the poll's actual findings.

For instance, regarding the finding that contraceptive-oriented sex-ed courses produce only a 40% rate of regular contraceptive use and are correlated with a greater number of students engaging in both contracepted and noncontracepted sexual intercourse, Planned Parenthood concluded that "education works!"[31] It is clear, though, that birth-control promoting sex-ed courses are correlated with 31% to 50% higher incidences of teen sexual intercourse, pregnancies, abortion, venereal disease, and the like. When Planned Parenthood terms this a "success," you have to stop and ask yourself just what its goals are.

---

31. Ibid., p. 56.

The experiences of other countries validate the conclusion that Planned Parenthood's birth control approach to sex education (and its emphasis on school-based sex clinics) is harmful to the sexual health of teens. A comparison of Sweden and the Netherlands is instructive:

> Sex education in Sweden is compulsory and extends to all grade levels. Information on contraception is provided, and there is a close link between the schools and teenage birth control clinics. No other country approaches this level of implementation. In the Netherlands, by contrast, sex education in the schools is limited to the teaching of reproductive biology. There is, however, a heavy emphasis on sex education in the mass media as well as public funding of educational efforts aimed at teens by private family planning associations.[32]

In addition, in Sweden, contraceptive services and supplies are free, but they are not free in the Netherlands.[33]

The disparate results of the two different approaches is dramatic. Sweden's level of teen sexual experience (ever had intercourse) is substantially higher than the Netherlands': about 60% higher at ages seventeen and eighteen. By age eighteen, more than 80% of Swedes have lost their virginity, and by age nineteen, about 90% have done so.

Despite the higher rates of sexual activity, one would expect Sweden to have the lower teen pregnancy rate due to its far greater emphasis on promoting contraceptive knowledge, usage, availability, and affordability. Alas, such is not the case. In fact, the teen pregnancy rate in the Netherlands is less than half the rate in Sweden. For instance, at age seventeen, about 1% of Dutch girls get pregnant, versus about 3% of Swedish girls; at age eighteen, the rates are 2% and 5%, respectively.

Obviously, Sweden's compulsory K-12 sex education promoting birth control usage, and its emphasis on providing free contraceptive services and prescriptions, has resulted in a far higher incidence of teen intercourse *and* teen pregnancy than that of the Netherlands, where the birth control approach is not employed.

---

32. Nadine B. Williams, ed., *Contraceptive Technology, 1986-1987*, (New York: Irvington Publishers, Inc., 1986), p. 26.

33. Ibid., pp. 25-26. Much of the discussion on Sweden and the Netherlands is drawn from this source.

The conclusions are clear: The main danger to teen chastity and to teen sexual health is a Planned Parenthood-style contraceptive-oriented sex indoctrination course.

It is interesting to note that Planned Parenthood's teen sex survey found that while amoral or immoral forms of sex education greatly worsen the problem of teen promiscuity and pregnancy, it also found that the single most effective way to reduce teen pregnancy seems to be moral education: Students who attended religious services frequently had a 53% lower rate of promiscuity than students who seldom or never attended religious services. It *is* true that education works, but *only* if it is traditional moral education.

The effect of religious education was enormous, greater than every other variable including race, education, economic status, scholastic achievement, gender, geographic location, the marital status or education of the parents, the students' future educational goals, whether their parents had discussed sex with them, or what type of sex education they received in school. Nothing, *nothing*, even came close to being as important as religious attendance in having an effect on teen sexual promiscuity.

And you know, the funny thing is that religious education *is* education. Yes, Planned Parenthood, education *is* the answer; education truly *is* the key to teen sexual behavior. If we want to increase the teen promiscuity problem by one-third to one-half, we merely need to implement comprehensive sex-ed programs. On the other hand, if we truly want to reduce the teen promiscuity problem by up to 53%, we should encourage frequent religious education.

Please remember that both Planned Parenthood Federation of America and affiliate Planned Parenthood clinics insist that sex education and religion are inseparably intertwined, that it is our religious beliefs that necessarily inform and influence our sexual behavior. Planned Parenthood has long asserted that sex education should be religious, indeed, is inescapably religious. Planned Parenthood has not been bashful at all about putting its destructive "fornication is-not-a-sin" sex-ed programs into our nation's public schools. And we should not be bashful or ashamed about insisting that our schools totally remove all vestiges of the "if-it's-right-for-you," Planned Parenthood-style sex-ed programs, and that they replace them with programs that reinforce the chaste, virginal lifestyles of the overwhelming majority of teens; which reduce peer pressure (far and away the leading cause of teen promiscuity); which emphasize the debilitating, incurable and sometimes fatal consequences of teen promiscuity; and which teach clear behavioral guidelines such as "say no to drugs" and "say no to premarital sexual intercourse."

It's funny: Schools can teach our children not to smoke pot, not to curse at the teacher, not to murder the principal, not to rape and beat their classmates, not to vandalize the gymnasium, not to rob the cafeteria cashier; but they can't bring themselves to give the students clear moral guidelines about sex outside of marriage. We don't give them choices about whether to murder the principal, but we leave it up to their own feelings and value systems to decide if they want to have sex with the teen sitting next to them. And then, when they have made a baby, we give them the choice of whether they want to have mercy on their poor, defenseless, innocent child or whether they would rather just have it murdered.

We cannot bring ourselves to tell our children not to have sex *because as parents we are less moral than our children.* Planned Parenthood's survey shows that kids are crying out to be told not to have sex. They're sick of the peer pressure. They're sick of having to sit in coed classes and talk about penises and vaginas and orgasms and semen and ejaculation and sperm and IUDs and diaphragms and oral sex and anal sex and on and on, day-after-day.

Teens are sick of having sex crammed down their throats by a wicked adult society. Teens don't want schools pushing birth control pills; they want schools pushing chastity. Eighty-eight percent of all teens do not want a school-based sex clinic in their school, and 79% think teens are having sex too soon. School-based sex clinics are dreaded by students because they represent just more peer pressure to cram sex and birth control pills down the throats of teens.

Teens are sick of being treated like animal-instinct idiots. They're sick of having sex and birth control shoved in their face by people who profit the most from teen promiscuity: Planned Parenthood clinics. They're sick of being treated like hopeless perverts mindlessly wandering through life in sexual ignorance, controlled totally by a few inches of flesh between their legs.

Teens are sick of being coerced into using contraceptives by being brainwashed in classes that only perpetuate the myth that "everyone's doing it." Teens are sick of being told that no one can catch AIDS by casual sexual contact, but that anyone, including chaste teens, can get pregnant or catch venereal diseases by casual contact.

Students are sick of having some antireligious course clarify their values. If schools were willing to risk transmitting some moral values, we would see students at far less risk for sexually transmitted diseases. Students are crying out for schools to put them at risk for morality instead of for AIDS and herpes. Planned Parenthood's study shows that what we teach puts them at risk for one or the other. What's worse? Is it really worse to have public school teachers tell your child that "fornication is a sin" than to have the school nurse tell him "you have AIDS"?

Planned Parenthood has mesmerized most of the establishment in America with its inherently racist arguments that comprehensive sex-ed courses, school-based sex clinics, and easy abortions are the cure to the problem of teen pregnancy, which Planned Parenthood claims is mainly a lower-class, minority problem. Planned Parenthood has used overt or implied racist appeals for over six decades now in order to gain white elitist establishment support for its birth control programs. The results of its 1986 teen sex survey were analyzed by race (white, black, and Hispanic — apparently no one has bothered to tell Planned Parenthood that Hispanic is not a *race*) so that Planned Parenthood would be able to make its standard blackmail appeal: Let us in to your schools or these low-class, indigent, uneducated minorities are going to overrun our schools and welfare system with more and more babies.

Despite its own overwhelming evidence to the contrary, Planned Parenthood still clings to the myth that amoral sex education is effective in fighting the moral problem of teen sexual immorality. In the foreword to its survey, Planned Parenthood says, "Sex education in the schools is the other way that society can break the cycle of low social status — low grades — low information about sexuality — low use of contraceptives — high risk of pregnancy."[34] But this supposed "cycle" does not exist at all, according to the survey.

---

34. Ibid., p. 8.

In fact, based on the results of Planned Parenthood's survey, there is a strong positive correlation between the level of a teen's sexual knowledge and his likelihood to have engaged in sexual intercourse. That is, low sexual knowledge is identified with low rates of sexual activity, while high rates of sexual knowledge are identified with high rates of sexual activity. This is exactly the opposite of the relationship that all sex education postulates.

Planned Parenthood and all sex educators insist that there is a negative, or inverse, correlation between sexual knowledge and sexual activity, or, at least, teen pregnancy. The belief that increasing teens' sexual knowledge can decrease their rates of fornication, and the incidence of teen pregnancy, abortion, and childbirth, is perhaps the most prevalent and most dangerous sexual myth in America today.

This is not to say that strictly biological sex education is correlated with higher rates of teen promiscuity. In fact, strictly biological sex education has repeatedly been shown either to have no effect on teen promiscuity or to result in a modest reduction in promiscuity. But Planned Parenthood is adamantly opposed to strictly biological approaches and to "moral" approaches to teen pregnancy. Planned Parenthood insists that only comprehensive, that is, birth-control-promoting, sex education courses are of any value.

Thanks to Planned Parenthood's 1986 survey, we have at our disposal the information we need to restore moral and practical sanity to our nation's schools. What remains is for us to rise up and do something about the crime of immoral, Planned Parenthood-style sex education. We need to break the *real* cycle of teen pregnancy:

> Young girl gets pregnant > Planned Parenthood hypes the need for contraceptive-oriented sex-ed > schools teach children how to have sex and use birth control > Planned Parenthood clinics give the girls "free" (taxpayer financed) birth control without their parents' consent > great increase in teen fornication and pregnancy > Planned Parenthood calls for even earlier amoral sex-ed in more schools, for school-based sex clinics, and for more government funding > cycle repeats itself.

PRESCRIPTION FOR DISASTER: TEEN-AGERS AND BIRTH CONTROL

Birth control as an accepted practice is a relatively recent phenomenon. In fact, no Christian denomination ever accepted any form of contraception as morally permissible for any reason before 1930, and the Catholic Church still forbids all methods of contraception except natural family planning, and then only for hard cases.[1] Yet birth control is the foundation of Planned Parenthood.

In fact, as the eugenics movement picked up steam worldwide in the late 1920s and early 1930s, led mainly by British and German eugenicists, the American birth control movement began to gain credibility too. Margaret Sanger, who is credited with having coined and popularized the term *birth control*, quickly allied her birth control efforts with this movement and outlined her goal "to produce a race of thoroughbreds."

Birth control quickly became, and still is, the foundation of Planned Parenthood. Sanger's birth control efforts had initially met stiff resistance from people concerned about "race suicide" because birth control practices were far more widespread among the upper-middle-class elite than among the working classes. However, with its new eugenic thrust, birth control became a popular upper-middle-class cause. The new thrust for birth control was to encourage its use by the "feebleminded," Jews, blacks, the poor, and any other class of citizens generally loathed or feared

1. John F. Kippley, *Birth Control and Christian Discipleship*, (Cincinnati: The Couple to Couple League for Natural Family Planning, 1985). The historical analysis presented here draws heavily on Kippley's work.

by the upper crust WASPs who were the main proponents of birth control.[2]

The first church to endorse birth control practices was the Church of England, in 1930, followed in America by the Federal Council of Churches, in 1931. Within thirty years, many churches had evolved from a grudging, conditional acceptance of birth control *in some circumstances*, to an outright endorsement and recommendation of birth control as a wholly Christian practice. Within less than fifty years, many churches even promoted abortion as a positive Christian action.

Even after birth control became an almost universally accepted practice, it was still primarily accepted only within the confines of marriage. *Until about 1960, even Planned Parenthood advocated limiting birth control use to married couples.* With the development and distribution of birth control pills in the very early 1960s, the pressure for releasing the remaining restrictions on the use of birth control by married and single persons greatly escalated.

In 1965, the Supreme Court bowed to the raging demands of the Sexual Revolution. In *Griswold v. Connecticut*, the Court invented a supposed constitutional "right to privacy" to justify striking down all barriers to the unrestricted use of contraceptives by married couples. Seven years later, it extended this newly created "right to privacy" to single persons, allowing them the same privileges as married persons in obtaining and using contraceptives.

Then, in 1973, the Supreme Court struck again. In *Roe v. Wade*, a lawsuit brought by a woman seeking to abort her child allegedly conceived in a gang rape,[3] the Court ruled that this "right to privacy" applied to abortion as well.

In the space of less than fifty years, birth control had gone from being widely rejected, to highly controversial, to widely accepted, and from illegal to a fundamental constitutional right. And with birth control came abortion.

That the legalization and acceptance of abortion should closely follow the legalization and acceptance of birth control was not

---

2. Linda Gordon, *Woman's Body, Woman's Right* (New York: Penguin Books, 1977). This analysis draws heavily from Gordon's very thorough research.

3. The Texas plaintiff known as Jane Roe admitted publicly in 1987 that she had fabricated the gang rape story that was the basis of *Roe v. Wade*. She was not raped.

coincidental—it was inevitable, because abortion is really just one method of birth control.

The terms *birth control* and *contraception* are often used interchangeably, but they do not mean the same thing. To practice birth control means to engage in practices to prevent the *birth* of a child, whereas to practice contraception means to engage in practices to prevent the *conception* of a child. Thus, birth control includes contraception, but it also includes practices to prevent the birth of a child after conception.[4] Obviously, birth control includes abortion as a method of preventing birth.

Similarly, family planning and birth control are two different concepts that are often used interchangeably. When Planned Parenthood says family planning, it always means a range of practices to limit the number of living children in a family, and these practices include abstinence, contraception, abortion, and sometimes, infanticide.

It is impossible to embrace the concept of family planning and reject the practice of abortion, for abortion is merely one tool of family planning. To say that you believe in family planning but reject abortion is as silly as saying you believe gardeners should avoid weeds but should not pull them out of their gardens.

The irony of birth control is not that it is so universally accepted, unquestioningly accepted, despite its relative infancy; the real irony is that birth control is so widely accepted despite being an antiquated, obsolescent concept, a totally outdated approach to the problem of teen fornication.

The concept of birth control is a dinosaur, a throwback to Stone Age days of hippies and pot and groovy tunes and nine-inch-wide paisley ties in fourteen shades of hot pink and electric blue and long sideburns two inches wide and Ward and June hoping the Beaver doesn't grow up to drop acid.

The concept of birth control should be relegated to the closet with the other eternal truths whose time has come and gone, truths like the earth is flat, marijuana makes you more creative, sodomy is a victimless crime, and Ronald Reagan can and will reduce the federal deficit.

---

4. For simplicity's sake, the terms *birth control* and *contraception* will be used more or less interchangeably throughout the text.

The fatal flaw in the concept of birth control is that it postu-lates pregnancy and childbirth as the only important undesirable results of fornication.

But they're not. And they never were.

To focus on pregnancy alone is to ignore the whole subject of venereal disease. From the discovery of penicillin until 1977 or so, ignoring venereal disease in a strategy to contain the fallout from sexual sin was a calculated gamble, but it was not a poten-tially *fatal* gamble.

After all, venereal disease was curable. And VD was nor-mally invisible, and if you got VD you didn't have to go to the venereal store and buy bigger clothes and waddle like a duck for nine months. Sure, VD was a nuisance, but penicillin was a swift, private, inexpensive, and guilt-free cure.

Until herpes. And until penicillin-resistant strains of gonor-rhea. And until they found that early sexual activity and multi-ple sexual partners greatly increase the risk of developing cer-vical cancer.

Still, the concept of birth control as a cure-all for the ills and hazards of unrestrained recreational sex retained its credibility and its near-universal approbation.

And then came AIDS. But AIDS was a gay disease: no limp wrist, no AIDS, right?

Wrong. AIDS is not a gay disease. AIDS is an incurable ve-nereal disease that is always fatal. AIDS makes a mockery of the right to privacy (maybe the Supreme Court will rule that AIDS is an unconstitutional intrusion) and of the concept of birth control.

The fundamental premise of birth control is that getting pregnant is bad. AIDS sets the record straight: The problem with fornication *is* fornication, not pregnancy.

The only truly safe and effective birth control device is a wedding ring dispensed at the local church, and the best method of family planning is to plan to have them with your wife. Unmarried minors do not need to be planning families. True family planning is a matter reserved for families (i.e., groups of people headed by Mom and Dad), and healthy families are not dispensed at Planned Parenthood in 28-day pill packets. The only appropriate oral contraceptive for unmarried teens is not the mini-pill; it's "NO."

No is always 100% effective. No is an appropriate method that can be used anytime, anywhere, by anybody. No not only prevents pregnancy and childbirth, it also prevents guilt, fear, worry, shame, emotional trauma, herpes, AIDS, syphilis, gonorrhea, chlamydia, venereal warts, and abortion.

But as we all know, No is a moralistic, preaching type of approach that just won't work with today's teens.

Wrong. That's the adult wisdom. The teens say otherwise.

The 1986 Louis Harris poll of American teens conducted for Planned Parenthood found that *79% of teens believe that most teens start having sex too soon.* It also found that the majority of teens say that "telling teens to worry about getting venereal disease" or "telling them how a pregnancy could ruin their life" or "telling them to worry about how their parents are going to react if they find out they're having sex" would be likely to influence teens to delay sexual intercourse.[5]

One of Planned Parenthood's questions in the poll was, "What do you think is about the right age for a person to start having sexual intercourse?" Planned Parenthood's entire philosophy of sex education is wrapped up in that one inane question. Planned Parenthood treats sexual intercourse as if it were a positive responsibility to be undertaken by teens as they grow up: "What do you think is about the right age for a person to start making up his bed? Helping his father mow the lawn? Tying his own shoes?"

Planned Parenthood phrases the question as if sexual intercourse were something teens ought to be doing if they would only grow up a bit. The utter depravity of Planned Parenthood's approach to teen sex can be discerned from its posing the question as a technical matter of age. By posing sexual intercourse as a technical matter of age, Planned Parenthood has already told teens that sexual intercourse is not a question of morality. Planned Parenthood should have asked whether teens considered sexual intercourse as acceptable outside of marriage, but that would have implied that sexual intercourse was a moral question. In fact, Planned Parenthood was so intent on avoiding the impression that sexual intercourse is a moral issue that it even declined

5. *American Teens Speak*, pp. 18, 60.

to ask, "What is the right age?" which might imply that there is a right answer. Instead, Planned Parenthood fuzzed up the question by making it a matter of personal feelings and approximate guesses: "What *do you think* is *about* the right age?"

Given the way the cards were stacked, it's surprising to see the answers given by the teens: Only 25% said that people under eighteen should ever have sexual intercourse, and only a minority said that any teen-agers should engage in sexual intercourse. Only 16% said that most teens wait long enough before they start having sexual intercourse.[6]

Nevertheless, the unquestioned assumption of adult society is that teens are sexual bohemians who have no moral values, and that we must therefore do whatever we can to encourage teen contraceptive use.

The foundational premise for pushing birth control to unmarried teens is that birth control is a safe and effective way to prevent pregnancy, and that all teens would use birth control if they could get birth control cheaply and easily. But birth control is neither safe nor effective in preventing teen pregnancy.

According to statistics published by the Alan Guttmacher Institute, birth control is not the cure for unmarried teen pregnancy. These are the actual in-use success rates for unmarried teens who use birth control: 7% who *always* use a prescription method of contraception will become pregnant within a year; 12% who *always* use a nonprescription method of contraception will become pregnant within a year.[7]

That means that a girl who faithfully uses prescription contraceptive methods through high school and college has a 44% likelihood of getting pregnant, and a 64% chance if she faithfully uses a nonprescription method (including a 25% chance of becoming pregnant more than once).[8] This is not a cure for out-of-wedlock pregnancy.

---

6. Ibid., p. 18.

7. Alan Guttmacher Institute, *Issues in Brief*, 4:3, (March, 1984). The Institute would probably disagree with my interpretation as to the meaning of these failure rates.

8. Ibid. Statistics were derived using the AGI first-year failure rates and extrapolating them over longer time intervals by using the binomial probability formula. This method probably underestimates actual contraceptive failure rates over extended time intervals because it ignores the deleterious effects of contraceptive method abandonment, method switching, and other factors.

The Alan Guttmacher Institute claims that 80% of all teen-agers who use contraceptives use prescription contraceptive methods.[9] Now, the above annual failure rates of 7% and 12% were for teens who *always* used birth control, and the most reliable data available shows that only 33% of sexually active teens who use birth control *always* use birth control.[10] Obviously, a lot of teens who are using birth control are getting pregnant, as the following analysis shows.

Analysis of Teen Pregnancy

In a letter to the editor of the *Wall Street Journal*, Planned Parenthood president Faye Wattleton displayed a rather typical example of the type of deliberate statistical misinformation that has characterized the hyping of the teen pregnancy crisis.[11] She said:

It is true, as Mr. Weed stated, that federally funded family planning clinics serve 1.5 million teenagers in the U.S. Yet he failed to mention that 11 million teenagers are sexually active and that 9.5 million sexually active teens remain unserved.[12]

The distortions in Mrs. Wattleton's statements are enormous. First, there are only about 29,000,000 teen-agers, and according to the results of the Planned Parenthood poll of American teens, only 28% of all teen-agers have had sexual intercourse. Thus, only about 8,120,000 American teenagers are sexually active, not 11,000,000. Mrs. Wattleton's estimate of 11,000,000 teens translates to 38% of all teens, a figure far higher than any reliable estimate.[13]

---

9. Ibid.

10. *American Teens Speak*, p. 19.

11. The pejorative term teen pregnancy is itself fraught with ideological bias, as the term tends to devalue pregnancies on the basis of the mother's age rather than her marital status. Use of teen pregnancy statistics without regard to marital status inflates the magnitude of the real problem: pregnancies to unmarried teens. See the chapter entitled "Teenage Pregnancy: Finding Solutions" for more discussion of the distortions and false assumptions inherent in the use of the term.

12. Faye Wattleton, letter to the editor of the *Wall Street Journal*, October 16, 1986.

13. A Planned Parenthood Federation of America "Fact Sheet" on teen pregnancy claims that there are 12 million sexually active teens.

Perhaps Mrs. Wattleton's greatest distortion involves her assertion that 9.5 million teens "remain unserved" because they do not patronize federally funded family planning clinics. First of all, of these 9.5 million "unserved" teens, 57% are completely unable to get pregnant because they are males.[14] Males do not patronize family planning clinics because males cannot use the Pill, diaphragms, or IUDs. The only nonsurgical male contraceptive is the condom, and condoms can be bought in drugstores and grocery stores and thousands of other places. There is absolutely no reason why any male would need to go to a family planning clinic or doctor's office to purchase condoms.

Faye Wattleton's remaining "unserved" population after subtracting the males would be about 3,250,000. But just because these girls do not frequent federally funded family planning clinics does not mean that they do not use birth control. In fact, according to the U.S. Bureau of the Census, sexually active women aged fifteen to nineteen average more than 1.5 annual family planning visits per person, a rate that is about 60% higher than for all other sexually active women.[15] About 55% of these women use family planning clinics (both private and government-funded), 39% use private physicians, and the remainder use counselors or other sources.[16] In all, about 79% of all sexually active teenage girls already use some method of birth control.[17]

Mrs. Wattleton also neglected to mention that of "11 million sexually active teenagers," about 7% are married, including about 611,000 females.[18] (About half of all births to teens are to teens who are married. For instance, in 1981 there were 536,000 births to women aged nineteen and under, but 268,000 of these births [50%] were to married women.)[19] Obviously, saying that 9.5

---

14. *American Teens Speak*, p. 16. About 32% of all teen-age boys have had sexual intercourse, versus 24% of all teen-age girls.

15. *Statistical Abstract of the United States: 1987*, no. 101, p. 67, 1982 data.

16. Ibid., p. 67.

17. *American Teens Speak*, p. 19.

18. From *Statistical Abstract of the United States: 1987*, no. 51, p. 41. 6.4% of all females fifteen to nineteen years old in 1982 were married, all of whom were presumed sexually active.

19. Compiled from *Statistical Abstract of the United States: 1987*, no. 86, p. 61 and unpublished data from the National Center for Health Statistics and the Alan Guttmacher Institute.

million sexually active teenagers do not frequent government funded family planning programs does not tell us much about how many teens are truly at risk for premarital pregnancy. So let's analyze the size of the at-risk population another way.

Of 11 million sexually active teens, only 4,730,000 are female and of these, 610,000 are married. This leaves 4,120,000 sexually active unmarried teen-age girls. But 79% of these sexually active teen-age girls use birth control,[20] *leaving only 865,000 sexually active unmarried teen-age girls who never use birth control. That's hardly "9.5 million at risk," is it?*

But even this at risk figure is probably too high, because these calculations were based on Mrs. Wattleton's exaggerated figure of 11 million sexually active teens. But using the more reliable, less exaggerated results of Planned Parenthood's 1986 teen sex poll, we can show:

> *There are 29,000,000 American teenagers;*
>   8,120,000 or 28% of these teens are nonvirgins;
>   3,490,000 or 43%, of these nonvirgins are girls;
>   610,000, or 17%, of these nonvirgin girls are married,
>   leaving 2,880,000 sexually active teen-age girls,
>   of which 2,276,000, or 79%, use birth control,
>   leaving a net figure of only 604,000 sexually active
>   American teen-age girls who never use birth control.

Thus, less than 3% of all American teens are unmarried sexually active teenage girls who never use birth control! This is hardly a crisis![21]

The implications of these statistics are enormous.

In order to reach 604,000 unmarried sexually active American teen-age girls who never use birth control, Mrs. Wattleton suggests the following program:

---

20. *American Teens Speak*, p. 19.

21. It is, however, a tragedy. Nevertheless, we do not live in the millennium or in a utopia. In every civilization that has ever existed (or that ever will exist), there have been at least some teens who have sex and get pregnant before marriage. Neither premarital sexual intercourse nor premarital pregnancy can ever be totally eradicated. The only realistic and sensible goal, therefore, is to hold the levels of premarital promiscuity and pregnancy down to the lowest residual level. The real crisis today is teen promiscuity, not teen failure to use birth control.

Parents must be helped to communicate earlier, more effectively and more consistently with their children about sexuality.
Television network officials must reverse their ban on contraceptive advertising and offer more balanced sexual program-
ming, including information about contraception. Local and
state policy makers must support sexuality education in every
school district, from kindergarten through twelfth grade, and
comprehensive school-linked health clinics that offer contraceptive information and services as part of general health care.
Federal officials must support a national initiative, broader
than the existing federal family planning program, to ensure
that primary prevention of teen pregnancy and elimination of
all barriers to family planning become national priorities.[22]

Parents *must*. Network officials *must*. Local and state policy
makers *must*. Federal officials *must*. Mrs. Wattleton has hyped
604,000 unmarried noncontracepting sexually active teens into a
crisis so severe that virtually every American must enlist in
Faye's army and do his part.

Notice that Mrs. Wattleton insists that Planned Parenthood-
style contraceptive-promoting sex indoctrination courses *must* be
administered to every American student, *starting with kindergartners*. How disgusting! The number of voluntarily sexually active
children under twelve years of age is statistically insignificant. A
substantial proportion of early sexual activity is caused by incest, and incest cannot be reduced by teaching kindergartners
about sex and birth control.

In fact, according to Planned Parenthood's poll, less than 10%
of all girls ages twelve to fourteen have ever had sexual intercourse.[23] *Pregnancies to girls under age fifteen are less than 0.5% of all
pregnancies (less than 2.5% of all teen pregnancies), and births to unmarried teens under age fifteen are less than 0.25% of all births (3.4% of
all births to unmarried teens).*[24] *Obviously if there is a teen pregnancy*

---

22. Faye Wattleton, letter to the editor of the *Wall Street Journal*, October
16, 1986. These proposals mimic the policies of Sweden. Sweden has the highest rate of teen sexual intercourse, higher than any other Western nation, including America, and the second highest abortion rate.

23. *American Teens Speak*, p. 15.

24. From National Center for Health Statistics, *Health, United States, 1986.*
DHHS Pub. No. (PHS) 87-1232, Public Health Service (Washington, D.C.:
U.S. Government Printing Office, December 1986), p. 23; and *Statistical
Abstract of the United States: 1987*, No. 84 and No. 86, pp. 60-61.

crisis, it doesn't start before age fifteen. Despite all of the Planned Parenthood-fostered hype regarding teen births, the birth rate for women ages fifteen to nineteen peaked in the late 1950s and has actually *declined* slightly since 1980 (it declined by 43% from 1960 to 1984).[25] And although the number of out-of-wedlock births to teens has increased by about one-third (because teenage girls are now far less likely to marry the father to legitimate the birth),[26] the teen birth rate and the annual total of teen births have declined substantially.[27] Why then does Faye Wattleton insist that Planned Parenthood-style sex indoctrination classes must start at age five? What's her real agenda?

Although Mrs. Wattleton's assertion that "9.5 million sexually active teens remain unserved" is a distortion designed to convey the false impression that millions of sexually active teenage girls are at risk for pregnancy because they are presently deprived of birth control services (which is as ridiculous as saying 200 million Americans remain unserved by medicine because they are not on Medicare), her statement does reveal much about Planned Parenthood's true agenda: to profit from teen fornication. It seems clear that Mrs. Wattleton's true concern is not "how many teens use birth control?" but "how many teens are clients of federally funded family planning clinics?"

Another incredible distortion by Mrs. Wattleton concerns the false implication that teen pregnancy can be eliminated by birth control. It cannot. In fact, the teen pregnancy crisis is

---

25. *Statistical Abstract of the United States: 1987*, no. 82, p. 59.

26. Alan Guttmacher Institute, *Issues in Brief* 4:2 (March, 1984); see also *Statistical Abstract of the United States, 1987*, No. 54, p. 42. The number of unmarried couples under twenty-five years of age increased over 750% from 1970 to 1985, and the number of unmarried couples with children under age fifteen more than tripled during that period. Charles Murray has documented in *Losing Ground* (New York: Basic Books, Inc., Publishers, 1984) that many government welfare programs contain strong economic disincentives to marriage, and may be partially responsible for substantial increases in unmarried cohabitation and the fathering of illegitimate offspring. Other studies have concluded otherwise. For instance, one study reports a negative correlation between high state AFDC payments and teenage birthrates. See, for example, Susheela Singh, "Adolescent Pregnancy in the United States: An Interstate Analysis," *Family Planning Perspectives* 18:5 (New York: Alan Guttmacher Institute, September/October, 1986).

27. *Statistical Abstract of the United States: 1987*, No. 82, p. 59.

caused by sexual intercourse and a failure *of* birth control, not by a failure to use birth control.

To illustrate this, we will analyze the source of teen pregnancies using three scenarios: (1) Faye Wattleton's overstated estimate of 11,000,000 sexually active teens, (2) Planned Parenthood's 1986 teen sex survey finding that 28% of teens are sexually active (i.e., 8,120,000 teens),[28] and (3) published data from the Alan Guttmacher Institute.

ANALYSIS OF THE SOURCE OF UNMARRIED TEEN PREGNANCIES

Scenario #1: Faye Wattleton's high estimate of 11,000,000 sexually active teens

> 29,000,000 American teens, of which
> 18,000,000 are virgins
> 11,000,000 are nonvirgins, of which
> 6,270,000 are males
> 4,730,000 are females, of which
> 610,000 are married
> 4,120,000 are single, of which
> 1,400,000 always use birth control
> 1,855,000 sometimes use birth control
> 865,000 never use birth control

Group	No. of Teens	Annual Probability of Pregnancy*	Pregnancies Per Year
Always use BC	1,400,000	8%	112,000
Sometimes use BC	1,855,000	24%	435,000
Never use BC	865,000	35%	303,000
	4,120,000	21%	850,000[29]

*The known annual pregnancy rates are 8% per year for single teens who always use birth control, and 35% per year for single teens who never use birth control. The "sometimes user" figures are necessarily plug figures calculated from the other known constraints.

Conclusion: In this scenario, 64% of all unmarried teen pregnancies are attributable to teens who use birth control, but not consistently or effectively.

---

28. *American Teens Speak*, p. 15.
29. The number of pregnancies per year to *unmarried* teens is about 850,000.

Scenario #2: Based on Planned Parenthood's 1986 teen sex poll finding that 28% of teens have had sexual intercourse

29,000,000 American teens, of which
20,880,000 are virgins
 8,120,000 are nonvirgins, of which
 4,630,000 are males
 3,490,000 are females, of which
   610,000 are married
 2,880,000 are single, of which
   980,000 always use birth control
 1,296,000 sometimes use birth control
   604,000 never use birth control

Group	No. of Teens	Annual Probability of Pregnancy*	Pregnancies Per Year
Always use BC	980,000	8%	78,000
Sometimes use BC	1,296,000	47%	560,000
Never use BC	604,000	35%	212,000
	2,880,000	30%	850,000[30]

*The known annual pregnancy rates are 8% per year for single teens who always use birth control, and 35% per year for single teens who never use birth control. The "sometimes user" figures are necessarily plug figures calculated from the other known constraints.

Conclusion: In this scenario, 75% of unmarried teen pregnancies are attributable to teens who use birth control, and two out of three pregnancies to unmarried teens are attributable to teens who use birth control, but not consistently or effectively.

Scenario #3: Data Published by the Alan Guttmacher Institute

According to data published by the Alan Guttmacher Institute, the 1976 and 1979 pregnancy statistics for metropolitan-area teens can be broken down as follows:[31]

---

30. See note 29.

31. Melvin Zelnick and John F. Kantner, "Sexual Activity, Contraceptive Use and Pregnancy Among Metropolitan-Area Teenagers: 1971-1979," *Family Planning Perspectives* 12:5 (New York: Alan Guttmacher Institute, September/October, 1980).

PERCENTAGE DISTRIBUTION OF WOMEN AGED 15-19 WHO EVER EXPERIENCED A PREMARITAL FIRST PREGNANCY, BY CONTRACEPTIVE-USE STATUS

Contraceptive-use status	1979	1976
Always used	14.0%	9.4%
Sometimes used	35.7%	31.8%
Never used	50.3%	58.8%
TOTAL	100.0%	100.0%

Conclusion: More than half of all pregnancies to metropolitan-area un-married fifteen- to nineteen-year-olds from 1976 to 1979 were attributable to birth control users.[32]

But something else happened between 1976 and 1979: there was a substantial increase in the rate of consistent birth control use, including use at first intercourse, and a substantial decline in the rate of never-use.[33] Never-use dropped 8.9 percentage points, to 26.6%, while always-use increased 5.5 percentage points, to 34.2%. These positive contraceptive trends should have produced a far lower teen pregnancy rate in 1979 than in 1976, but they didn't: In fact, as contraceptive usage increased significantly, the rate of pregnancy among fifteen- to nineteen-year-olds rose substantially, by 8.2%.[34] And in 1979, 13.5% of unmarried female teens aged fifteen to nineteen who always used birth control reported that they had gotten pregnant, as well as 30% of teens who sometimes used birth control.[35]

Obviously, efforts to persuade more teens to use birth control were successful in persuading more teens to begin having sex, but not to use consistent contraception. *All of the increase in metropolitan-*

---

32. Ibid., from table 8, p. 236. Most pregnancies from 1976 to 1979 would have to be attributable to birth control users in order to lower the proportion attributable to never users to 50.3% from 58.8%.

33. Alan Guttmacher Institute, *Teenage Pregnancy: The Problem That Hasn't Gone Away*, 1981, p. 11.

34. See Stanley K. Henshaw, "U.S. Teenage Pregnancy Statistics," (New York: Alan Guttmacher Institute, September, 1986).

35. Melvin Zelnick and John F. Kantner, "Sexual Activity, Contraceptive Use and Pregnancy Among Metropolitan-Area Teenagers: 1971-1979," *Family Planning Perspectives* 12:5 (New York: Alan Guttmacher Institute, September/October, 1980).

area teen pregnancy from 1976 to 1979 was attributable to teens who were birth control users:[36]

PERCENTAGE INCREASE IN METROPOLITAN AREA TEEN PREGNANCIES, 1976-1979, BY CONTRACEPTIVE-USE STATUS

Source of Teen Pregnancy	Percentage Increase
Those teens who:	
Always Use Birth Control	+ 59.9%
Sometimes Use Birth Control	+ 20.6%
Never Use Birth Control	− 8.1%

Teens and Contraception

The advocates of the birth control approach to the teen pregnancy problem assume that there is some magic method for turning sexually irresponsible teens into 100% responsible contraceptors. No such magic method exists.

In fact, to raise teens' contraceptive usage even minimally requires a tremendous amount of persuasion and preaching about birth control. Teens are remarkably resistant to practicing effective contraception. *Even after taking a Planned Parenthood-style comprehensive sex indoctrination course, only 40% of sexually active teens will practice contraception all the time.*[37] That means that, at best, 60% of all sexually active teens will remain at very high risk for pregnancy, while 40% will have *at least* an 8% *per year* risk of pregnancy.[38]

---

36. Computed using statistics on the percentage distribution of metropolitan-area women aged fifteen to nineteen who ever experienced a premarital first pregnancy, by contraceptive-use status, 1976 and 1979, and assuming that these percentages can be applied to the fifteen- to nineteen-year-old pregnancy rates for those respective years. This assumption results in an approximation, but certainly the results are very close to the mark. Computing the percentage increases using only the cumulative percentages and ignoring the absolute changes in the level of teen pregnancies results in the following figures for the respective categories: Always users, up 48.9%; Sometimes users, up 12.3%; Never users, down 14.5%. The result is substantially the same, perhaps slightly more dramatic.

37. *American Teens Speak*, p. 7.

38. Weighted average of prescription and non-prescription contraceptive failure rates for unmarried teens who always use contraception, as found in Alan Guttmacher Institute, *Issues in Brief* 4:3 (March, 1984).

The *net* effect of efforts to persuade or enable teens to use contraception is to aggravate the teen pregnancy problem by increasing the number of teens who are sexually active, including the number of teens who are sexually active but do not use effective contraception or any at all. (Of course, the term *effective contraception* is a gross misnomer when you consider that a teen-age girl faithfully practicing "safe sex" [her boy friend using condoms] has about an 18% per year chance of getting pregnant, and a 64% chance over a five-year span of at least one pregnancy.)[39]

Even if we could get *all* sexually active teens to practice "safe sex," the number of teen pregnancies per year due to contraceptive failure would be *at least* 630,000 (assuming no increase in the number of sexually active teens, a ridiculously unrealistic assumption). But just to raise the percentage of sexually active teens who regularly practice contraception to 40% (not 100%), we would probably see an increase in the level of teen pregnancies of 10% to 30%.[40]

Birth Control Failure Rates

We've wanted to believe in birth control because we wanted to believe that there could be a painless technical solution to the moral problem of teen fornication. But birth control is what has put an entire generation at risk for AIDS by pretending that the only undesirable result of fornication is pregnancy. Ask an AIDS victim about the dangers of fornication—I doubt pregnancy will rank high on the list.

We simply must educate teens and society that birth control methods do not render fornication "safe." Not even barrier methods

---

39. William R. Grady, Mark D. Hayward, and Junichi Yagi, "Contraceptive Failure in the United States: Estimates for the 1982 National Survey of Family Growth," *Family Planning Perspectives* 18:5 (New York: Alan Guttmacher Institute, September/October, 1986), p. 204; one-year failure rates were extrapolated over longer intervals using the binomial probability formula. Because the effectiveness of any contraceptive method drops as coital frequency and period of use increase, this method of calculating multiple-year failure rates may understate contraceptive failure.

40. See Myth 10 in the Chalkboard Evangelists chapter.

such as condoms can transform God-cursed fornication into "safe sex." Nor does contraception prevent pregnancy; it merely delays it.

Here are the actual in-use failure rates for various methods of birth control for single women:[41]

IN-USE CONTRACEPTIVE
FAILURE RATES FOR
SINGLE WOMEN

Method of Contraception	Annual Risk of Pregnancy
Pill	5.9%
Diaphragm	23.3%
IUD	5.4%
Condoms	10.8%
Rhythm	23.0%
Spermicides	19.4%
Withdrawal, other	15.4%
No Method	44.7%

As you can see, the effectiveness rates of the diaphragm (a prescription method) and of the rhythm method (a nonprescription method) are almost identical. It should be noted that these failure rates are averages; for persons who are more than normally active sexually, these failure rates are understated.[42]

But these failure rates by no means tell the whole story. In order to see the real failure of birth control, we need to look at the cumulative probability of getting pregnant over longer time periods, because the value of a birth control method depends on its ability to continuously prevent pregnancy.[43]

---

41. William R. Grady, Mark D. Hayward, and Junichi Yagi, "Contraceptive Failure in the United States: Estimates for the 1982 National Survey of Family Growth," *Family Planning Perspectives* 18:5 (New York: Alan Guttmacher Institute, September/October 1986), p. 204.

42. Ibid.

43. Ibid., p. 204. The five-year and ten-year rates shown have been derived by this author using the binomial probability formula to extrapolate AGI's published first-year failure rates over extended intervals.

CUMULATIVE PROBABILITY OF PREGNANCY FOR SINGLE WOMEN BY METHOD OF BIRTH CONTROL

Method of Contraception	Chance of at Least One Pregnancy			Chance of at Least Two Pregnancies	
	1 yr	5 yr	10 yr	5 yr	10 yr
Pill	6%	25%	44%	3%	11%
Diaphragm	23%	73%	93%	33%	72%
IUD	5%	24%	43%	3%	10%
Condoms	11%	44%	68%	9%	29%
Rhythm	23%	73%	93%	33%	71%
Spermicides	19%	66%	88%	25%	61%
Withdrawal, Other	15%	57%	81%	17%	47%
No Method	45%	95%	99%	74%	98%

Obviously, birth control does not prevent unintended pregnancies; used long enough, it virtually assures them. And condoms are hardly "safe sex" facilitators: *about half of unmarried condom users will have at least one pregnancy within a five-year period.*

But these failure rates are for single women of all childbearing ages. The failure rates for unmarried teen-age girls are far higher, roughly twice as high:[44]

IN-USE CONTRACEPTIVE FAILURE RATES FOR TEEN-AGE GIRLS UNDER 18 WHO ARE TRYING TO PREVENT A PREGNANCY

Method of Contraception	Annual Failure Rate
Pill	11.0 %
Diaphragm	31.6 %
IUD	10.5 %
Condoms	18.4 %
Rhythm	33.9 %
Spermicides	34.0 %
Other	21.1 %
No method	62.9 %

Again, we can extrapolate these failure rates over longer time intervals to derive a more relevant measure of contraceptive failure:

---

44. Ibid., table 5.

CUMULATIVE PROBABILITY OF PREGNANCY FOR TEEN-AGE GIRLS UNDER 18 WHO ARE TRYING TO PREVENT A PREGNANCY BY METHOD OF BIRTH CONTROL

(in percent, results rounded to whole numbers)

Method of Contraception	Chance of at Least One Pregnancy			Chance of at Least Two Pregnancies	
	1 yr	5 yr	10 yr	5 yr	10 yr
Pill	11%	44%	69%	10%	30%
Diaphragm	32%	87%	98%	50%	87%
IUD	11%	43%	67%	9%	28%
Condoms	18%	64%	87%	23%	57%
Rhythm	34%	87%	98%	55%	90%
Spermicides	34%	87%	98%	55%	90%
Other	21%	69%	91%	29%	66%
No Method	63%	99%	99%	93%	99%

You can bet your life that these figures would come as a total shock to virtually all of the sexually active teens who have taken a Planned Parenthood-style sex education course or who have received birth control at a Planned Parenthood clinic. Unfortunately, these teens are being fooled into a false security that using birth control can effectively prevent pregnancy and (in the case of condoms) venereal disease — and these deceived teens are the ones who are betting their lives, and the lives of their about-to-be-conceived children.

Clearly, the high-risk group for pregnancy and venereal disease is unmarried teens who have sex, not teens who do not use birth control. A fifteen-year-old girl who has sex and uses condoms has a 68% to 87% chance of getting pregnant at least once by age twenty-five, and a 29% to 57% chance of two or more pregnancies. So much for "safe sex." On the other hand, a fifteen-year-old girl who does not have sex until she marries at age twenty-five has no chance of pregnancy or venereal disease.

Pregnancy is the result of sexual intercourse, whether contracepted or not. People who have sexual intercourse will get pregnant eventually; it's all just a matter of time. Birth control does not prevent pregnancies, it merely makes pregnancy somewhat less likely in any given time frame, compared to noncontracepted intercourse.

Let's take another example: a fifteen-year-old girl who decides to use condoms but who will not marry until age thirty-five because of her career ambitions. This girl has the following likelihood of premarital pregnancy:[45]

Cumulative # of pregnancies	Likelihood of pregnancy
none	10%
1 or more	90%
2 or more	65%
3 or more	37%
4 or more	16%
5 or more	6%

Why are condoms so ineffective? Well, one reason is that condom users sometimes fail to use condoms in the heat of passion. And some condoms break and some condoms slip off. But another real problem is that condoms have a remarkably high rate of defects. In their 1965 book entitled *Planned Parenthood, A Practical Guide to Birth-Control Methods*, Abraham Stone and Norman Hines insisted that modern condoms were very safe:[46]

> When condoms varied greatly in quality, it was advisable to test each condom individually before use. Techniques for inflating the condom like a balloon with air, filling it with water or testing it with cigarette smoke were recommended. With current methods of manufacture and testing by the producers and the rigid quality control exercised by the Food and Drug Administration, such testing by the users has become unnecessary and even dangerous; clumsy manipulation during testing may actually start small cracks or holes in the latex and predispose the condom to rupture during coitus.

Stone and Hines expressed complete faith in the quality of modern condoms:

---

45. Extrapolating the first-year failure rate of 10.8% for all single women who use condoms over a twenty-year interval using the binomial probability formula. See footnote 28 in Chapter 2.

46. Abraham Stone and Norman Hines, *Planned Parenthood* (New York: 1965), pp. 197, 200.

If it is to be preserved for future use, the condom should be soaked in water, otherwise it is likely to dry out during the night and tear when pulled apart. It should be washed thoroughly, filled with water, and turned inside out several times under flowing water. The use of a mild soap is advisable but not necessary. After it is dried on both sides with a towel, it should be dusted with French chalk, cornstarch or ordinary talcum powder. *There is no reason why a condom of good quality cannot be used six to ten times.* (italics added)

Six to ten times? The U.S. Food and Drug Administration believes that many modern condoms should not be used *even once*:

One of every five batches of condoms tested in a government inspection program over the last four months failed to meet minimum standards for leaks, according to the U.S. Food and Drug Administration, which called the failure rate unexpectedly high.

At the same time, ongoing laboratory research in both the United States and Canada has already led to the conclusion that lambskin condoms allow the leakage of the AIDS, herpes, and hepatitis B viruses.

And in a report published last week, a Department of Health and Human Services task force concluded that "there are no clinical (human trial) data supporting the value of condoms" in preventing the spread of a range of diseases, including syphilis, herpes, hepatitis B, and human immunodeficiency virus, the precursor of AIDS.

Together, those developments underscore broadening concern about some of the premises of the condom mania sweeping the United States in response to the AIDS crisis. The reliance on condoms as an AIDS protection has escalated, even though the condom was never designed or manufactured to control sexually transmitted diseases.

At the University of Southern California, Dr. Gerald Bernstein, who is working on a government-funded condom evaluation, summed up: "Using condoms is not really what people are talking about when they say safe sex. It may be safer sex, but I think it's a misnomer to say condoms are safe sex."[47]

---

47. "Many Condoms flunk FDA's test for leakage," *The Houston Chronicle*, August 20, 1987.

Despite the overwhelming evidence, Planned Parenthood continues to insist that condoms render fornication safe from pregnancy and venereal disease and AIDS. And, of course, Planned Parenthood continues to equip the overwhelming majority of fornicators with nonbarrier contraceptive methods, dooming them to herpes, AIDS, and pregnancy.

Summary

We must return to the simple truth that pregnancy is the result of intercourse rather than a failure to use birth control. The major cause of teen pregnancy is the failure *of* birth control, not a failure to ever use birth control.[48]

Planned Parenthood's hype regarding teen pregnancy has fostered the false belief that almost all teen pregnancies are attributable to teens who never use birth control. That is false. Only one in four American teen-age girls has ever had sexual intercourse, and of the girls who have, only 21% never use birth control. The number of sexually active, unmarried American teen-age girls who never use birth control is less than 3% of all teenagers. Given these statistics, it is not surprising to find that the majority of pregnancies to unmarried teens are attributable to birth control users.

The birth control approach to teen pregnancy is unrealistic. It can never hope to lower teen pregnancy rates without a substantial amount of coercion, because sexually irresponsible teens are also sexually irresponsible contraceptors.

But the failure of teen contraception is not limited to irresponsible contraceptive behavior by teen birth control users; unfortunately, there is also a core group of teen-agers who are sexually active but who do not want to use birth control because they simply "prefer not to" or because they feel birth control destroys the spontaneous, unplanned nature of their sexual exploits.

Because teens' failure to reliably use contraception is largely rooted in human nature, efforts to raise teens' contraceptive usage

---

48. Ninety-five percent of all American women of childbearing age have used some method of birth control, and 76% have used the Pill. See, for example, National Center for Health Statistics, W. D. Mosher and C. A. Bachrach: Contraceptive Use, United States, 1982, *Vital and Health Statistics*, series 23, no. 12, p. 25.

are predictably futile. In fact, efforts to raise teens' contraceptive usage are *counterproductive*: increases in teens' voluntary use of contraceptives have resulted in increases in teen pregnancies because those efforts have been more successful at convincing teens to have sex than to use birth control consistently.

The birth control approach to premarital pregnancy is also unrealistic because it has encouraged a tremendous rise in long-term premarital sexual activity, which has itself put tremendous strains on the ability of birth control to prevent premarital pregnancy. And contraceptive failure rates have been tremendously understated by stressing theoretical failure rates and failure rates over meaninglessly short time periods such as one year.

For a fifteen-year-old girl, neither the theoretical failure rate nor the one-year failure rate for the diaphragm is relevant. Girls don't use birth control in a biological textbook; they use it in the real world. Teen-agers don't get pregnant in theory, they get pregnant in the real world. And the relevant contraceptive failure rate for a fifteen-year-old girl is not the one-year failure rate; it's probably the five-year rate, maybe the ten-year rate. A fifteen-year-old diaphragm user has more than a 75% chance of getting pregnant at least once by age twenty. Birth control is hardly the solution.

Unfortunately, too many Americans refuse to face the facts about teen pregnancy. For too many, contraception just seems like common sense: You're less likely to get pregnant if you use contraception. What most people have not grasped is that what makes sense on a one-to-one basis does not work on a macro scale. If we could somehow isolate just sexually active teens and persuade *them* to use contraception, we could probably lower the teen pregnancy rate. But we can't do that. We can't identify and isolate teens who have had premarital sex, and we can't persuade *all* sexually active teens to *always* use birth control. What makes sense is clearly unworkable; there's just no practical way to do it, short of coercion (ask the Chinese).

The "get-'em-on-birth-control" approach cannot be implemented on an as-needed, one-to-one basis, but neither can it be implemented on a macro scale. Increasing teens' use of birth control *increases* teen pregnancy.

Unfortunately, Planned Parenthood continues to ignore the fact that teen-agers' usage of contraceptives cannot be increased without worsening the teen promiscuity rates. However, a recent study in *Family Planning Perspectives*, published by Planned Parenthood's research arm, shows just how ineffective birth control really is in fighting the tragedy of teen pregnancy.[49]

According to this study, if we were able to cut sexually active unmarried American teen-agers' nonuse of contraception in half, teen pregnancy would fall by only 27%. For both married and unmarried teenagers as a whole, a 50% decrease in nonuse of contraception would cut teen pregnancy by only 20%:[50]

> For both black and white teenagers, [the model] assumes a 50 percent increase in the use of the pill, at least a doubling of condom use, a slight increase in the use of remaining methods and a 50 percent decline in nonuse. . . . Such a shift implies a modest reduction of 20% in the unintended pregnancy rate.[51]

Obviously, even if we could eliminate half of noncontracepted teen sexual intercourse, we could still make barely a dent in teen pregnancy. There would still be at least 900,000 teen pregnancies per year.

Even if we were able to totally eliminate contraceptive nonuse among unmarried American teens, so that all teens who had sexual intercourse always used contraception, we would reduce the incidence of unmarried teen pregnancy by less than one-third.[52]

Of course, even these slight reductions are completely unattainable, as the study admits:

---

49. Charles F. Westoff, "Contraceptive Paths Toward the Reduction of Unintended Pregnancy and Abortion," *Family Planning Perspectives* 20:1 (New York: Alan Guttmacher Institute, January/February 1988), pp. 4-13.

50. Ignoring the fact that increases in contraceptive usage can only come at the expense of more teen promiscuity; any projected reduction in teen pregnancy due to increased contraceptive utilization would be wiped out by a great increase in the number of teens who were sexually active.

51. Ibid, p. 9.

52. Ibid, p. 10.

This is a quite unrealistic projection for both age-groups, however, since some non-use will persist, and, of course, pill use will not increase as much as these numbers would suggest.[53]

But the study also ignores the fact that any significant increase in contraceptive usage among unmarried American teenagers, if it is attainable at all, will come only at the expense of a significant increase in both the percentage of teens who are sexually active, and in coital frequency among sexually active teens; both of these factors would wipe out any gains from increased contraceptive usage.

The evidence is overwhelming that the birth control approach to teen pregnancy does not work, has not worked, and will not work. Birth control is more than just a flawed approach to the moral problem of premarital promiscuity; with the advent of AIDS and herpes and other incurable venereal diseases, the birth control approach is outdated, in fact, deadly.

It's time to face the facts.

---

53. Ibid, p. 10.

RUBBER SOUL:
THE HYPOCRISY
OF "SAFE SEX"

Planned Parenthood often insists that it wants to see fewer teen pregnancies, yet Planned Parenthood is the foremost proponent of, and supplier for, teen promiscuity. Why? Because Planned Parenthood is a master at promoting its own programs as the solution to the very problems they create.

While publicly insisting that it wants to reduce teen pregnancy and abortion, Planned Parenthood hypocritically promotes the notion of "safe sex," fostering the perception that sex outside of marriage can be both safe and responsible.

Consider this contradictory posture by an analogy: that of the local drug pusher. The local drug pusher insists that taking drugs is a victimless crime and that young people (and older people) take drugs for a variety of reasons, including peer pressure, to relieve stress, to experiment and satisfy natural curiosity, because it feels good, and many others. He points out that drug use has always existed and that virtually everyone uses some drugs: aspirin or caffeine or alcohol or cocaine.

The drug pusher says he believes that many teen-agers begin to use drugs and then get into trouble because of a real lack of knowledge about drugs. He quotes surveys that show that many of the students have real misconceptions and ignorance about drugs and what they do ("12% of the students think you can get high by shooting mayonnaise, and 28% think that you can't get high the first time you smoke marijuana"). The pusher also points out that many drug users are harmed by an inability to obtain (or, in some cases, *afford*) safe drug supplies, free from harmful contaminants.

So, to show his real concern for teen-age drug abuse, the pusher proposes a two-pronged program to the local school board. He proposes a new course to be taught to all students, starting in the sixth grade, to inform them about all the different types of illegal drugs that are available and about their effects, both pleasurable effects and some of the possible complications. Not using illegal drugs will be presented as one option, but the course will concentrate on how to use drugs safely rather than on abstaining from drug use.

Some of the main points of the course are:

1. Not using illegal drugs is an option. But not using illegal drugs cannot guarantee 100% safety from becoming a drug bum because there is always the chance that you might have a bad reaction to a legal medication, or someone might slip LSD into your Kool-Aid.

2. *Anyone* can become a drug bum. Lots of very famous and very talented people were drug bums.

3. Some people use drugs responsibly and safely.

4. If you do use drugs, never share needles, and always use a pure drug supply.

5. No one can tell you when *you* are ready to use illegal drugs; you must make your own decision.

6. If you are going to use illegal drugs, or you suspect you are already a drug bum, go to a well-respected local drug pusher who can help you get a safe drug supply and learn to use it responsibly.

The drug pusher goes on to suggest that the school may even want to consider establishing a school-based drug clinic where students can go to talk with a sympathetic professional about drugs and drug problems and where they can get a safe drug supply and learn to use it responsibly.

Swell guy, isn't he? The community's most prolific drug pusher has the gall to suggest that he is a vital part of helping school children avoid becoming drug bums.

Well, the drug pusher is Planned Parenthood. And the drug is the contraceptive, and sometimes abortifacient, Pill. Substitute promiscuity for illegal drug usage and the Pill for illegal drugs and you have the current scenario.

Planned Parenthood is not interested in eliminating teen promiscuity; it is interested in promoting teen promiscuity and profiting from it.

So when the AIDS crisis loomed ever more threatening in late 1986, Planned Parenthood perceived both a real threat and a golden opportunity. A real threat, because AIDS threatened to put the "fear of God" into a lot of sexual hedonists; and a real opportunity, because Planned Parenthood sensed that once again, it could promote its own programs as the solution to another promiscuity crisis.

And so almost overnight, Planned Parenthood became the messenger of latex salvation, spreading the good news to legions of fearful sexual bohemians that promiscuity and sodomy could indeed be "safe sex." Whereas once, Planned Parenthood had virtually scorned the prophet from Troy and trumpeted the superior graces of the chemical queen, in a flash of time, Planned Parenthood converted to the new faith, and clung to the hope in a new and better way: barrier methods.

And what zealous faith Planned Parenthood had! All across the land, Planned Parenthood began to speak rapturously of the miracles wrought by thin latex walls: AIDS viruses stopped dead in their tracks; deadly bodily fluids repelled effortlessly; inconvenient pregnancies completely averted. And the best news of all was that you didn't have to give up the old pleasures, the old lecherous habits. Yes, the new latex savior would accept you just as you are, and you wouldn't lose any of that good feeling you used to get doing it the old way.

But to the unsaved, the new faith seemed more than a little irrational. First of all, the new preachers were insisting that ritualistic condom usage provided complete protection against AIDS, herpes, sperm, blood, feces, urine, and anything and everything else. You almost expected them to say it could also cure the common cold and improve digestion. One got the distinct impression that it was almost safer to fornicate *cum* condom than to abstain from sex *sans* condom.

Not everyone was sold on the efficacy of the new latex salvation. The uninitiated found it hard to believe that the lowly condom was now held in such high regard. After all, was it not Planned Parenthood that had spent the last twenty-five years reminding us that the condom was only 85% to 90% effective in actual usage due to leaks, tears, breaks, slippage, overflow, incompatibility with lubricants, and failure to interrupt spontaneity to faithfully perform the ritual?

Besides, sometimes the preachers said "condom" when they really meant just the latex type and not the kinds that were made from sheep intestines. Everyone knew that the sacrificial lambs had yielded a product that was actually porous to the AIDS virus, and yet the messengers of the new salvation often confused the hearers by failing to make distinctions between latex condoms and processed sheep intestines.

Theologically, Planned Parenthood had always been most comfortable with the birth control pill. The Pill was a liberating device; it equipped women for the same sort of consequence-free (or seemingly so) sex that men had always enjoyed.

The Pill was also the best device for facilitating spontaneous, thoughtless sex. The Pill was taken routinely, daily, regardless of whether sex was contemplated, so it freed women from the tyranny of the shame and guilt that often came with having to stop and plan for contraception before engaging in sex. And the Pill never interfered with the pure sensual pleasure of it all—it required no foams, no lubricants, no artificial barriers or coverings.

In short, the Pill was ideal: liberatingly routine, but irreversible (on a daily basis), and solely dependent upon the woman for its effectiveness. Little wonder, then, that the Pill had always been promoted as the *primo* birth control form, the weapon of choice in the war on sperm.

By contrast, the condom had always been seen by Planned Parenthood as better than nothing, but not a lot better. The condom enslaved women to the voluntary cooperation of men, cooperation that sometimes required an awkward type of urging before it was grudgingly adopted for use by the man.

The condom was also a real bummer to use. Planned Parenthood deeply believed in the value of carefree, spontaneous sex, and the condom represented anything but spontaneity. Unlike the Pill, the condom could be employed effectively only after sexual arousal had already occurred, and its consistent use therefore required both a good deal of self-control and a willingness to substitute deliberation for spontaneity.

Besides the theological inadequacies of the condom, it also suffered as a method of contraception from a far greater failure rate. The actual in-use failure rate for all Pill users was about five pregnancies per year, while for condom users the rate was maybe three times as high.

Perhaps the only saving grace of the condom was that it did afford some protection against venereal disease transmission. Plus, it was affordable and readily available to minors. But then again, Planned Parenthood and Title X made the Pill readily available to minors, too, and venereal disease was curable.

Genital warts, herpes and antibiotic-resistant strains of syphilis and gonorrhea should have changed the equation, but their devastating effects went unheeded and Planned Parenthood continued to push the Pill as "protection" for unmarried fornicators. Ironically, the Pill not only left women totally exposed to all manner of venereal diseases, but it actually worked to lower women's natural resistance to some venereal diseases.[1]

Even though AIDS had gained national attention back in 1981, it wasn't until late 1986 that it became widely understood that AIDS was a venereal disease and, as such, a threat not only to the practice of promiscuity, but also to fornicators themselves. Almost overnight, AIDS threatened to unravel all of the perverse "gains" of the Sexual Revolution and drive sexual intercourse back into the confines of monogamous marriage.

Planned Parenthood could no longer afford to pretend that AIDS was so extremely hard to acquire. Even as late as early 1987, Planned Parenthood affiliates often insisted that AIDS was communicable only by massive exchanges of blood, semen, or feces, and that perversions such as fellatio or cunnilingus were probably safe.

---

1. See, for example, Robert A. Hatcher, M.D., et al, *Contraceptive Technology 1986-1987*, 13th revised edition.(New York: Irvington Publishers, Inc., 1986) p. 139 and others. The authors summarize the problem as follows: "Unlike condoms or diaphragms, oral contraceptives (OC's) provide no physical barrier to the transmission of sexually transmitted diseases (STD's). OC's have, in fact, been linked by some to increasing STD rates by (1) causing abandonment of barrier methods and (2) leading to increased sexual activity. . . . [E]pidemiologic and biologic evidence seems to indicate that infection with Chlamydia trachomatis is enhanced by oral contraceptives."

The masses didn't buy it: The average Joe in Peoria did not appreciate being labeled as homophobic or hysterical just because he refused to stick his head in the sand and pretend that an incurable, fatal, venereal plague could be fought by education — "if you're not sure, use a condom." The masses refused to buy the concept of homosexuality rendered antiseptically safe by the skillful application of a few latex socks.

The average John and Mary on the street weren't the only ones who refused to buy into the new "safe sex" theology: As with any new sect, apostates and heretics soon sprang up. Ed Koch, the liberal, prohomosexual mayor of New York City, instructed the City Health Department in early 1987 to revise its newly developed AIDS education materials to stress abstinence as the only truly safe protection from AIDS. Koch insisted that condoms were definitely not safe, and he forbade the City Health Department from promoting them instead of abstinence.

The defectors from the "safe sex" theology were not limited to political figures. In June 1987, the *Houston Chronicle* published a lengthy op-ed essay by Rice University professor James R. Thompson, an expert in statistics and biomathematics, who used historical, medical, and mathematical evidence to show that promoting the "safe sex" theology and downplaying the gruesome and very real threat of AIDS was actually fostering its spread.

The essay pointed out that AIDS is a venereal disease spread by infected parties, and that the best way to stop the spread of such a disease is to reduce the numbers of people likely to have sex with infected people, and to reduce the number of contacts of the most prolific carriers. The best way to reduce the incidence of casual AIDS-prone sex is to allow AIDS hysteria to run unchecked, Thompson asserted, because as people get deathly afraid of contracting an invisible, incurable, invariably fatal venereal disease, they will forsake the perverse sexual activities that transmit the disease.

Planned Parenthood's own poll of teen sex practices found that fear of the grave consequences of promiscuity would be effective in reducing teen promiscuity, but Planned Parenthood's version of the fear tactic is a predictable perversion of the one cited by teens. Planned Parenthood minimizes the negative consequences of teen promiscuity, but exaggerates the negative consequences of teen childbirth. Planned Parenthood has twisted the "fear" tactic into a way to generate more abortion business rather than using proper education to dissuade unmarried minors from engaging in sexual intercourse.

By downplaying the risks of unmarried sex, and by ridiculing AIDS fears as "hysteria," the "safe sex" evangelists have actually contributed to the continued growth of this plague. The advocates of "safe sex" were never really interested in stopping AIDS, though; primarily, they were interested in protecting the survival of the Sexual Revolution, and secondarily, hoping to slow the spread of AIDS.

If Planned Parenthood truly believed that only ritualistic condom usage could baptize promiscuity and render it safe, then it certainly did not act like it. While AIDS raged, Planned Parenthood continued to counsel young teen-age girls that intercourse was a responsible choice, and it continued to equip them with the Pill and other unsafe birth control methods without their parents' consent or advice.

According to the PPHSET clinic visit records, of 377 women who relied on condoms as their birth control method before they visited PPHSET, 280 were unmarried and therefore at increased risk for AIDS.[2] After visiting PPHSET, 252 of these unmarried women no longer used condoms as their primary birth control method; most had been converted to dependence on the Pill, which provides no protection whatsoever from AIDS or any other venereal disease.

On the other hand, PPHSET did persuade 174 unmarried people (out of 5,715) to use condoms. Most of these 174 people had been using no contraception at all. Even if you could just net the two sets of statistics (and you can't justify killing one person with AIDS just because you might have saved his neighbor from the disease), PPHSET was still a net dissuader of condom usage: A net 78 unmarried people were dissuaded from condom usage.

But the real statistics lie in percentages. We can see just how little PPHSET practiced what it preached by looking at likelihoods: A client walking into PPHSET that used no birth control

---

2. These statistics are drawn from this author's analysis of 6000 PPHSET Clinic visit records.

method or a method other than condoms had only a 4.4% chance of being a condom user at the end of the visit, while a condom user entering the clinic had only a 11.7% likelihood of remaining so at the end of the visit. *In other words, PPHSET equipped 95.6% of its clients to use life-threatening, nonbarrier birth control methods, and it persuaded 88.3% of its clients who use "safe" methods to quit doing so.*

If unmarried sex without condoms is unsafe, then Planned Parenthood is endangering the lives of its unmarried clients by offering them birth control methods that provide no protection whatsoever against AIDS, herpes, or any other venereal disease. For instance, of 2,145 women who were Pill users before they came to PPHSET, 178 were administered pregnancy tests, and 49 were actually diagnosed as pregnant (of these 49 pregnant Pill users, none were referred for adoption).

Of 377 condom users, 62 received pregnancy tests and 24 of these were diagnosed as pregnant. In all, out of 2,953 contraceptive users who visited PPHSET, 314 were administered pregnancy tests and 104 were diagnosed as pregnant.

A fertile female is capable of conceiving only a few days per month; however, venereal disease can be transmitted at any time. Thus, we would expect venereal disease transmission to occur at a relatively higher rate than contraceptive failure. Of 2,953 clients who were contraceptive users, 1,221 underwent venereal disease diagnosis or treatment. The figures for repeat patients (patients who were seen by PPHSET at least once before in the previous twelve months) are even worse: of 3,270 total repeat patients, 535 were seen for pregnancy tests, 333 were diagnosed as pregnant or suspected of being pregnant, 65 had abortions or were referred for abortions, and 1,255 were subjected to venereal disease diagnosis or treatment.

Despite what Planned Parenthood believes, promiscuity begets many varied negative consequences, including psychological afflictions, venereal diseases, pregnancy out of wedlock, and death. Thus, to isolate pregnancy as the sole negative consequence to be avoided is shallow and irrational. As the AIDS and herpes and chlamydia epidemics have shown, pretending that promiscuity and other perverse sexual practices can be safe or responsible will not and cannot remove God's curse from sexual sin.

And it is clear that much of the responsibility for the spread of AIDS within the heterosexual population rests with Planned Parenthood, which has stressed unsafe prescription (nonbarrier) methods of contraception over the safer and cheaper and more readily available barrier method. Nationally, 80% of the clients at family planning clinics receive prescription contraceptives.[3] Apparently, Planned Parenthood believes that "safe sex" is a lot less important than free sex.

It is naive to think that government-funded family planning clinics will ever willingly forego dispensing prescription contraceptives to unmarried women. To do so would be to commit organizational suicide: Dispensing condoms rather than birth control pills and IUDs and diaphragms would decimate Planned Parenthood clinics' revenues and profits. No pelvic exam or fitting procedure is needed to equip women with nonprescription, barrier-method contraceptives.

If condoms are truly the only method for "safe sex," then taxpayers should not be forced to support the dispensing of unsafe, expensive, nonbarrier contraceptives by Planned Parenthood or any other organization. Indeed, such a policy is not only wasteful and misguided, but a direct threat to the health of the client and of the nation as a whole. Clearly, the federal government must, at minimum, quit subsidizing the contraceptive abuse and exploitation of unmarried women by family planning clinics. Since it is unrealistic to expect Planned Parenthood clinics to commit organizational and economic suicide by promoting condom usage, it is clear that the most realistic way to encourage condom usage is to eliminate taxpayer funding of family planning clinics.

---

3. *Organized Family Planning Services in the United States, 1981-1983* (New York: Alan Guttmacher Institute, December 1984), p. 5.

SAFE AND LEGAL: THE NIGHTMARE OF LEGAL ABORTION

"Get her up and get another in here. Let's go, let's go, come on, goddammit." Dr. Kleberg was in one of his foul, unpredictable moods again. This time he was taking it out on the patients as well as the staff.

Dr. Kleberg hated Friday afternoon clinics anyway, but this afternoon was especially irritating. The women were all supposed to be prepped and ready to go in rapid fire by 4:30, and here it was 4:55 and he had only gotten one done and he had twelve more to go, and he needed to be home by 6:30 if he ever expected to make the cocktail party, and then here's this ignorant fool of a patient ("f---ing patients," he usually called them, with more than a touch of irony intended) who refused to move after he had finished the procedure.

Dr. Kleberg had been fairly cheerful starting Marcia's "procedure" even though the staff had been unable to sterilize all of the instruments from the morning abortions with Dr. Leerson, and they hadn't been able to start until 4:45. Dr. Kleberg and Marcia seemed to hit it off just fine, and after he had removed the cannula from her uterus she had said that "it really wasn't bad at all."

And now she wouldn't move. Marcia simply refused to make any effort to get up at all. She just laid there frozenlike looking really put out, and not answering questions or responding to the nurse's pleas for her to sit up.

Dr. Kleberg had finally asked her to "please get up," to no avail, and now he was starting to lose his cool.

"Get that thirteen-year-old in here, *now!*" he barked. "And get this idiot off the table and into the recovery room whether she likes it or not."

The nurse (they called her a "VPT Aide" at the clinic; VPT stood for "Voluntary Pregnancy Termination," which sounded better than "abortion" although no one could ever *prove* that any of the babies had volunteered to be "terminated") held the little girl's hand as she escorted her into the killing room. Nicole was scared, *very* scared, and the fact that her father had brought her there for the abortion didn't make things any better.

Nicole was not sure that she was ready for a baby, but she was certainly not sure that she was ready for an *abortion*. Nicole wasn't ready to have sexual intercourse, either, but no one had ever bothered to tell her that. She wished she were about five years older so she could just go ahead and get married and have the baby. But Nicole's dad had never even considered any course of action, except that she was going to have an abortion, period.

It's funny, thought Nicole, how young girls who have sex are treated like adults, and how young girls who have abortions are treated like adults, but how young girls who want to birth their babies are treated like children. Every woman has a right to an abortion, they say, but no little girl has the right to have a baby.

Nicole had heard Dr. Kleberg yelling, but she couldn't hear what he was saying. All she knew is that he looked really angry when she walked into the room, and the woman lying like a stiff on the other table didn't exactly put her at ease.

Nicole was really embarrassed by the thought of having this strange man putting his hands and his machines into her private parts. The pelvic exam the nurse had given her earlier to confirm the pregnancy was bad enough, but the thought of this strange man putting a suction tube up through her cervix gave her chills.

Nicole had been so absorbed in her fears that she really hadn't paid attention to what anyone was saying to her. Dr. Kleberg's overpowering volume broke her trance. "You better hold still or I'm not going to do you," he barked at the quivering little girl.

Marcia, meanwhile had been escorted into the recovery room by two assistant VPT Aides. She had begun moaning, and she continued to moan in recovery for over an hour, to the great consternation of the clinic staff who kept checking her every fifteen minutes and insisting that she was well enough to leave. The VPT Aide remarked that she had *never* seen anyone take so long to go through the clinic.

Does Legal Mean Safe?

The advocates of child butchery are fond of telling us that thanks to *Roe v. Wade* abortion is now safe and legal. They tell us about the "millions of women who died from back alley abortions," and they cite statistics that show that very early abortions are now safer than childbearing (when measured in total deaths).

But Roe v. Wade didn't outlaw back alley abortions; it legalized them.

Overnight, what had once been a heinous crime became legal. The back alley baby butcher no longer had to conceal his operation; he was now immune to prosecution. Effective January 22, 1973, back alley abortions in America became *legal* back alley abortions. The back alley butchers hung out signs and starting taking credit cards. (What do *you* think happened? You think the back alley butchers gave it up when it became legal?)

Legalizing abortion couldn't, and didn't, make it safe. Abortion, whether officially sanctioned or officially proscribed, always kills women and children. Every abortion is fatal to at least one person, the child, and some abortions, legal or not, are fatal to both the mother and the child. The purpose of abortion is to snuff out innocent life; that's hardly safe.

The actual number of women who were dying per year from abortion, legal or illegal, immediately prior to 1973 was probably about 250 per year. That's the hardly millions of women that abortion advocates claim were victimized by abortion before 1973. But abortion is still dangerous, and now, after fifteen years of "safe, legal abortion," abortion is the sixth leading cause of maternal death. And, abortion deaths are probably under-reported by at least 50%.

Organizations such as Planned Parenthood and the National Abortion Federation quote statistics that purport to show that very early abortions are safer than childbirth. Murdering a defenseless, powerless, nameless victim may be safe for the murderer; it certainly is not for the victim. And just because murdering defenseless people may be safer than certain kinds of self-sacrificing charity doesn't mean that we should encourage murder and discourage charity.

Just because certain illegal acts may be rendered safer for the perpetrators by making them legal does not give us sufficient grounds to legalize them. Abortion is murder, and although not all murder can be stopped by good laws and good law enforcement, we still need laws against murder; and we still need swift prosecution of murderers. Legalizing rape might make rape safer for rapists, but to legalize rape would be itself a horrible crime.

The whole concept of safety for inherently criminal, vile, ungodly acts like abortion and rape is begging the question. Safety is not the highest ethical standard in life. Do we legalize selling drugs to schoolchildren to ensure that they get a *safe, legal* drug supply? ("They're going to do it anyway," you know.) Do we legalize rape to make it less brutal for the woman and less dangerous for the rapist? ("You can't legislate morality," you know.)

Do we legalize sodomy to make homosexuality less emotionally devastating for the homosexual? America already tried that—and now, thanks to our misplaced mercy upon a whole generation of homosexuals, we have condemned both them and tens of thousands of innocent victims to die the slow, cursed death of AIDS.

Safety is not the highest ethical standard, and it is not a reliable standard for formulating or repealing moral laws. We in America have forsaken good concepts like righteousness and holiness and justice and tried to make our law too merciful.

But the primary purpose for law has never been to show mercy. Ultimately justice and mercy are contradictory goals. The role of civil government is not to operate as an agency of mercy; that mission properly belongs to the Church. But because the American church is so weak, so self-centered, and so lacking in basic ministries of mercy to the poor, the alien, the widow, and the fatherless, Americans have understandably sought to convert the State into an agency of mercy as well as justice. And so, we have sought to change the laws so as to make them more merciful.

We legalized and liberalized divorce laws in order to have mercy on spouses trapped in bad marriages that they were unwilling to fix; we legalized sodomy in order not to offend the poor perverts who delight in anal intercourse; we abolished capital punishment for most capital crimes in order to show compassion for the poor criminals trapped in a life of violent crime because of their environment; and we legalized abortional killing to show mercy upon the mothers who refused to defend the defenseless.

The results of our blasphemous attempts to be more merciful than God give evidence of the folly of our endeavor. Liberalizing divorce didn't save the family; it wrecked the family. We refused to enforce the laws against sodomy, and as a result we condemned untold thousands of innocents to die from contaminated transfusions, and sometimes, casual, routine daily contact — health care professionals infected by such means as accidental needle pricks. Similarly, our abundant mercy for those who commit capital crimes led to a rise in capital crime: Innocent people died because we had mercy for the wrong people. And lastly, in order to show our compassion for a relatively few women who might die while trying to murder their children, we condemned tens of millions of unborn persons to death by tearing, cutting, burning, and suffocation.

We cannot be more merciful than God. God's laws may seem strict, but they are fair. However, our standards of mercy and justice have been defective, unfairly one-sided. We have failed to comprehend the whole picture, to consider the innocent as well as the guilty. We have evaluated our laws primarily in light of their effect. upon the guilty and the criminal rather than upon the innocent.

This defective standard is readily apparent in the ludicrous argument that legal abortion is *safe*. Safe for whom? Safe for the guilty, or safe for the innocent? When one out of every three new Americans is murdered in a "legal" abortion, we can hardly call abortion *"safe."*

Nevertheless, organizations such as Planned Parenthood continue to spread the good news that a legal abortion is a safe abortion. But is it?

The scenarios depicted in the beginning of this chapter are dramatized composite accounts of actual incidents recorded in a small sample of abortion documents recovered from a Planned Parenthood clinic. An analysis of the available ninety-two abortion records dispels the notion of "safe" and "compassionate" abortion.

Of ninety-two women who had abortions, thirty-six were described as having been in severe or very severe pain. In addition, three women were said to have screamed during the killing procedure, while ten cried during the procedure, five were "complaining," and nine "overreacted." After the procedure, six women vomited or had nausea and six fainted.

The documents show an extreme callousness toward the mothers. In one abortion file, the doctor's disregard for the mother's health and safety is described by the VPT Aide:

> Dr. Leerson started the procedure without sterile gloves. He inserted the sterile speculum, clamped the uterus & then did the g.c. He literally crammed the cannula in, withdrew it upon seeing the pain she was in and gave her a block. — I think his sterile procedure should be questioned.

Ah, safe, legal abortion.

Dr. Leerson is described in another file as having recommended and performed an abortion for a girl whose pregnancy test gave a negative (not pregnant) result, on the grounds that it would relieve her anxiety. Two other files appear to be abortions on women who were not pregnant, although that seems not to have been known before the abortion. *The doctor was tipped off by the fact that the suction jar contained only tissue rather than fragments of a baby.*

These ninety-two abortion records reveal the real disdain the clinic personnel hold for the women who get abortions. Women who do not display the requisite amount of ambivalence or grief or trauma or regret seem to provoke a disgusted reaction from the VPT Aide. For instance:

> Apathetic towards her future and her past — left her child with people in Arkansas. Doesn't know where she'll be tomorrow. Very talkative, carefree. Doesn't seem to want any responsibilities. Will probably not be too conscientious about birth control. Seemed to be a rather confused young lady. No problems concerning decision or during procedure.

> *   *   *

> Very apathetic. Not concerned at all about birth control or repeated abortions (or financial situation). Made wisecracks in VPT room and laughed at inappropriate moments. Unaffected by entire procedure.

> *   *   *

> Attitude too casual about VPTs. May be a typical repeater. Tried to have a really tough attitude.

The pattern is unmistakable: The Planned Parenthood staff are bothered by women who truly buy in to their rhetoric about how abortion is a harmless, safe, legal, wonderful procedure with no complications, emotional or physical.

The abortionist and the staff are bothered by flippancy because they of all people know that murdering babies is nothing to be flippant about.

Mothers who are flippant about their abortions cheapen and devalue the work that the staff want so desperately to see as compassionate and merciful and necessary. Abortion may be murder, but it's necessary, compassionate, merciful murder, they believe. To the staff, the mother's psychological anguish as she confronts the horror of sacrificing her own child, and then decides that she must go through with the abortion anyway, becomes a redemptive ritual.

To the staff, their bloody work is sanctified by the mother's "brave" decision to commit murder even though it involves great emotional anguish and permanent loss. The staff become heroes in their own eyes as they seek to help women carry out the most guilt-ridden decision of their lives. Women who refuse to express such sentiments are despised because they transform the killing staff from heroic agents of aid, mercy, and compassion into mere accomplices to murder, hired killers.

Thus, the staff recoil with disgust whenever they are confronted with one of these women who view their abortions as little more than a trifling inconvenience. Women who thoughtlessly obtain repeat abortions are especially despised. An abortion in which the baby's death is greatly mourned by the mother is a valuable abortion: The worth of the abortion outweighed the worth of the baby's life. But an abortion in which the mother refuses to acknowledge the presence or humanity or worth or loss of the baby is a worthless abortion, a senseless and unjustifiable waste of human life. Such is the mentality of the killing staff.

The following pages contain verbatim[1] excerpts from these 92 actual Planned Parenthood abortion files, detailing in the participants' own words the gruesome callousness of abortional killing.

---

1. In the interest of readability, the patient information data has been put into paragraph form.

Name: Gladys P.

Patient information: Single, no children, but wants children. Has not been using contraception, but intends to get on the Pill after the abortion.

Before abortion: Talkative, tense.

During abortion: Screamed, overreacted, complained. Mild pain.

After abortion: Weak, tried to vomit.

Observations: Gladys and her boyfriend questioned the complications very vehemently. They asked about risk of death several times. Before the VPT, Gladys said she was going to scream and vomit and told her boyfriend she may never see him again. In procedure room, she tensed up and wiggled when Dr. Fredricks washed her off. She started to scream and moan during VPT but I told her not to. After VPT, she gagged several times when Dr. Fredricks examined her. After she got out of VPT room she seemed to recover quickly. Had a lot of support from boyfriend. Was scared to take Pill, but consented.

Name: Donna S.

Patient information: Divorced, one child. Wants more children. Used the Pill for one year. Has not used the Pill for two years. Intends to go back on the Pill after the abortion.

Before abortion: Relaxed, talkative, sense of humor.

During abortion: No pain.

After abortion: Walked.

Observations: Apathetic towards her future and her past — left her child with people in Arkansas. Doesn't know where she'll be tomorrow. Very talkative. Carefree. Doesn't seem to want any responsibilities. Will probably not be too conscientious about birth control. Seemed to be a rather confused young lady. No problems concerning decision or during procedure.

Name: Gail R.

Patient information: Single, Baptist, no children. Wants children. Using spermicidal foam and the rhythm method. Intends to use the Pill after abortion.

Before abortion: Nervous, realistic.

During abortion: Mild pain.

After abortion: Walked.

Observations: Excellent patient. Pregnancy test was negative today (not first specimen), but Dr. Leerson did not feel she should put off the VPT. Either way he felt it would relieve anxiety. Gail was given the choice to wait or have VPT done and decided to go ahead with VPT. She seemed a little upset, but decision was firm. Nice girl!

Name: Sherry S.

Patient information: Single, Methodist, no children. Does want children. Used the Pill for six months, but it caused nausea. Not presently using contraception.

Before abortion: Relaxed, realistic, talkative.

During abortion: Pain was severe at times.

After abortion: Walked.

Observations: Very mature 17-year-old. Good birth control attitude, but lots of side effects from Pill. I think she will make a real effort to take the Pill. Mother is very supportive and realistic about Sherry. She will be fine.

Name: Cecilia S.

Patient information: Divorced, Catholic, one child. Not sure if she wants more. Used the Pill off and on for five years (obtained Pill from Planned Parenthood), but the Pill made her nauseous. Presently using condoms; was using a condom when she got pregnant. Will continue to use foam and condoms after the abortion.

Before abortion: Tense, nervous, complaining. Cried.

During abortion: Mild pain.

After abortion: Walked, cried.

Observations: Would not relax at all—Dr. Wall very patient—Cecilia cried and jumped around—had more mental anguish than any physical reactions—could it be Catholic feelings? She wanted to stop for a minute right when Dr. Wall inserted cannula but Dr. Wall said he couldn't wait. Procedure went fine but after Cecilia got dressed, she cried and complained unjustly about Dr. Wall being rude and impatient. He was never rude. She was just taking out her feelings on the doctor. I explained why he proceeded with VPT when she asked him to wait. She left unhappy with doctor but she was calmed down and more rational. Cecilia was jittery during group and was fairly vocal. When I talked with her before VPT, she was nervous, but her decision was firm and did not consider other alternatives. Background and personal problems probably added to her reaction to Dr. Wall. Also, this seemed to be an outlet for her emotions about the VPT. Once this is behind her I think she'll do okay. Attitude toward birth control: *Very bad.*

Name: Rita P.

Patient information: Single, Baptist, no children. Does not use contraceptives, but will take Pill after the abortion.

Before abortion: Tense, quiet.

During abortion: Pain was severe at times.

After abortion: Weak, vomited.

Observations: Would not recognize need for birth control. Taking Pills only to "regulate her period." Very frail, thin, quiet little girl. Mother accompanied Rita and provided good, but not overpowering, support. Left question of birth control up to Rita. Appeared to be good relationship. Rita left with a smile!

Name: Donna P.

Patient information: Married, Roman Catholic, no children, but wants some. Has used the Pill and IUD, but Pill caused fluid retention and lumps in legs, and IUD caused excessive bleeding and cramping. Has been using diaphragm for two months.

Before abortion: Tense, nervous, talkative.

During abortion: Pain was severe at times.

After abortion: Weak.

Observations: Was nervous and was cramping hard after the procedure. Much better when she left. . . . very calm about repeat procedure. Was painful but she came through great!

Name: Laura S.

Patient information: Single, no children. Not sure if she wants any children. Uses spermicidal foam and the rhythm method.

Before abortion: Nervous, tense, sense of humor.

During abortion: Mild pain.

After abortion: Walked.

Observations: Seemed pretty nervous — laughed at inappropriate times. Left hurriedly after procedure. Good support from mother.

Name: Lauraine S.

Patient information: Single, Catholic, no children. Wants children. Uses contraceptive foam. Will use the Pill after the abortion.

Before abortion: Realistic, some nervousness.

During abortion: Mild pain.

After abortion: Walked.

Observations:

Editor's Comment: She used the Pill for three years, missed some, got pregnant and had a second abortion.

Name: Lauraine S.

Patient information: Single, Catholic, no children. Wants children. Uses the Pill, but missed some before she got pregnant. Started using the Pill after her first abortion at Planned Parenthood three years ago. Will continue the Pill after the abortion.

Before abortion: Relaxed, realistic, talkative.

During abortion: Mild pain.

After abortion: Walked. Talkative.

Observations: Excellent patient. Abortion almost too easy.

Name: Chrystal R.

Patient information: Single, Catholic, no children. Wants children. Used the Pill for one year, but legs ached. Was using IUD when she got pregnant.

Before abortion: Tense, nervous, quiet.

During abortion: Mild pain.

After abortion: Walked.

Observations: No problems noted with the decision.

Name: Edith P.

Patient information: Single, no children, but does want children. Former Pill user, now uses spermicides. Was using foam when she got pregnant.

Before abortion: Tense, realistic, talkative.

During abortion: Pain was severe at times.

After abortion: Fainted.

Observations: I asked Edith if she was ready to get up and she said she was. I had my arm around her shoulder and my other arm was placed on her arm. She started pulling away from me and fainted. She hit her head on the wall, but came to quickly. She asked if she fainted, smiled and said she was all right. She didn't get up any sooner than normal from the table. She was, however, a large person and too heavy for me to hold. She was fine in the recovery room and all smiles in the TV room. Note: Dr. Hinson present when she fell—he used ammonia ampule —BB.

Name: Azza S.

Patient information: Married, Moslem, one child. Wants more children. Used the Pill, but developed ovarian cyst. Presently using condoms and was using condoms when she got pregnant.

Before abortion:

During abortion:

After abortion:

Observations: Azza was a good patient and had a good attitude. Dr. F thought she might not be pregnant or very early since very little tissue was obtained. Urge her to come back for two week exam! Received in recovery room via wheelchair.

Name: Deborah S.

Patient information: Single, Christian, no children. Does want children. Uses the Pill, but missed some last month. Will continue to use the Pill after the abortion.

Before abortion: Overreacted, talkative.

During abortion: Pain was severe at times. Moist clammy skin. Hyperventilating; encouraged slow deep breathing.

After abortion: Weak.

Observations: She and Dr. Porter got along well. Then she really complained about the pain after saying, "It wasn't bad at all." She would make no effort to get up afterwards. Dr. Porter did another procedure and had to wait until we moved her. She moaned in recovery and was in there for over one hour. She felt like she was being rushed, but I've never seen anyone take as long to go through the clinic.

Name: Marianne S.

Patient information: Single, Baptist, no children. Does not want children. Uses the rhythm method, but wants to get sterilized or take the Pill after the abortion.

Before abortion: Overreacted. Cried, screamed, tense, nervous, complaining.

During abortion: Pain was severe to very severe.

After abortion: Talkative.

Observations: Very much overreacted. Very immature in every way. She was taking diet pills and seemed to be wound up. Kept insisting on getting a LAP and being a career woman. Agreed to take Pills but I'm not sure she will take them very long since she is sure she will gain on them. Attitude toward birth control: *very questionable.*

Editor's Comment: This was her second abortion. She used the Pill and foam and condoms for a year and then got pregnant and had her third abortion at Planned Parenthood.

Name: Marianne S.

Patient information: Single, Baptist, no children. Does not want children. Uses foam, condoms, and the Pill. Got pregnant while using condoms and the Pill. Intends to keep using the Pill after the abortion. Says she will take the Pill religiously from now on.

Before abortion: Overreacted, complaining, talkative.

During abortion: Pain was mild.

After abortion: Talkative, walked.

Observations: Received in recovery room via wheelchair. Severe cramping, colon good. She's sweet—but she simply does not understand and cannot comprehend that a method has to be used correctly in order for it to work. Attitude toward birth control: *extremely poor*!

Editor's Comment: This was her third abortion in three years.

Name: Janell S.

Patient information: Married, member of First Christian Church, one child. Does not want any more children. Used the Pill for five years. Planned Parenthood fitted her for an IUD; used it for six years. Developed uterine cancer—had half of uterus removed. Presently not using contraception, but will go back on the Pill after the abortion.

Before abortion: Talkative, nervous, cried.

During abortion: Pain was severe at times.

After abortion: Walked, talkative.

Observations: To recovery room appearing in good spirits; Dr. Leerson said she had a conization possibly but uterus intact! This woman is a very confused sick woman. She is one hundred pounds overweight but that is only a small part of her problem. Husband is alcoholic and the twelve-year-old son must have real problems. She says she is a child psychologist (with fifteen years education), truck driver, horsewoman, dog breeder, and on and on. Just an incredible talker (incessant). Needs constant attention. May have imaginary problems.

Name: Evelyn P.

Patient information: Single, no children, but wants children. Used the Pill for one year, but discontinued use due to amenorrhea. IUD user for one and a half years; had IUD removed after conception. Will have IUD re-inserted after abortion.

Before abortion: Tense, cried, nervous, talkative.

During abortion: Mild pain. Over-anticipated what was to happen — actually had no problems.

After abortion: Walked

Observations: No problems noted with decision. Crying seemed appropriate.

Name: Marsha P.

Patient information: Single, no children. Doesn't want any. Used the Pill for five years, but presently uses nothing. Intends to get back on the Pill after the abortion.

Before abortion: Tense, screamed, overreacted.

During abortion: Pain was severe at times.

After abortion: Weak.

Observations: Marsha is a "reformed" drug addict. She may have trouble staying on her birth control pills. She screamed and moaned throughout procedure — was extremely tense from GC to last pelvic exam — terrible patient, but nice lady. Received patient in recovery room via wheelchair and appeared in satisfactory condition.

Name: Suzanne S.

Patient information: Single, Methodist, no children. Does not want children. Has not used contraception, but will take the Pill after the abortion.

Before abortion: Realistic.

During abortion: Pain was very severe.

After abortion: Weak.

Observations: The procedure took thirty minutes. Dr. Hinson did a D&C. It was painful for Suzanne, but she did beautifully. She became very weak and her hands were stiff. The jar was half full of blood and I'm relieved nothing serious happened — it was that involved.

Name: Aurelia R.

Patient information: Single, Catholic, no children, but wants children. Does not use contraceptives, but will go on the Pill after the abortion.

Before abortion: Quiet

During abortion: Mild pain.

After abortion: Walked.

Observations: Has possible venereal disease. Speaks Spanish only. Asked her permission to tell her aunt and she agreed. Her aunt is going to take her to Central Health and I feel she understands the gravity of the situation.

Name: Nancy P.

Patient information: Married, two children, does not want more children. Former Pill user. Pill caused breakthrough bleeding and headaches. Uses a diaphragm; was using condoms when she got pregnant. Believes that after the abortion, she will be "happy and content with my two children I have."

Before abortion: Tense, realistic, talkative, sense of humor.

During abortion: Pain was severe at times.

After abortion: Walked, talkative.

Observations: Dr. Leerson started the procedure without sterile gloves. He inserted the sterile speculum, clamped the uterus & then did the g.c. He literally crammed the cannula in, withdrew it upon seeing the pain she was in and gave her a block. — I think his sterile procedure should be questioned.

Name: Consuelo R.

Patient information: Single, Catholic, one child. Wants more children. Does not use contraception, but will go on the Pill after the abortion.

Before abortion: Some nervousness.

During abortion: Tense, quiet.

After abortion: Walked.

Observations:

Editor's Comment: Planned Parenthood prescribed the Pill after the abortion. She used the Pill for eight months, but stopped using it because she did not like it. She got pregnant again about two years later and had a second abortion at Planned Parenthood. Once again, they prescribed the Pill. However, Consuelo was considered to have a "terrible" attitude toward birth control. She indicated she might switch to a diaphragm later.

Name: Consuelo R.

Patient information: Single, Catholic, one child. Wants more children. Had an abortion at Planned Parenthood. They prescribed the Pill. Used it for eight months, then dropped it. Got pregnant two years later. Intends to go back on the Pill only temporarily after the abortion. May switch to the diaphragm.

Before abortion: Tense, nervous, quiet.

During abortion: None to mild pain.

After abortion: Walked.

Observations: Consuelo jumped during procedure and tore the cervix — extra bleeding occurred. Dr. P. said it was OK and would heal soon. To recovery room by wheelchair. No distress noted. Terrible patient! Very negative about pills — may consider a diaphragm later.

Name: Gail B.

Patient information: Married, Catholic, two children. Wants more children. Used the Pill for four years, but was using spermicidal foam when she got pregnant. Intends to switch back to the Pill after the abortion.

Before abortion: Tense, nervous, realistic.

During abortion: Pain was severe at times.

After abortion: Walked.

Observations: Procedure was very long. Dr. Leerson had to use forceps to get some of the tissue. Gail was very tense and in a great deal of pain at times but recovered quickly. Left VPT room with a smile! Nice realistic lady.

Name: Shane P.

Patient information: Single, religious preference is "metaphysics," no children, but wants children. Has never had contraception, but will take the Pill after the abortion.

Before abortion: Nervous, talkative.

During abortion: Mild pain.

After abortion: Weak.

Observations: Mature attitude — she will be fine.

Name: Shane P.

Patient information: Single, no children. Wants children. Got pregnant while using the Pill. She had an abortion here about eight months ago, and they prescribed birth control pills for her. They thought her attitude toward birth control was "good," but the Pills ran out in six months and she did not bother to get a refill.

Before abortion: Relaxed, realistic, talkative.

During abortion: Mild pain.

After abortion: Walked, talkative.

Observations: Attitude too casual about VPTs. May be a typical repeater. Tried to have a really tough attitude. Attitude toward birth control: *fair — not serious.*

Name: Connie S.

Patient information: Single, member of Assembly of God, no children, but does want children. Has not used contraception. Wants to go on the Pill after the abortion.

Before abortion: Tense.

During abortion: Pain was severe at times.

After abortion: Weak.

Observations:

Editor's Comment: She went on the Pill for one and a half years, but the Pill made her sick, so she quit taking it. She got pregnant again and had her second abortion at Planned Parenthood.

Name: Connie S.

Patient information: Single, member of Assembly of God, no children. Wants children. Used the Pill off and on for eighteen months after her first abortion at Planned Parenthood, but the Pill made her sick. Had already discontinued Pill use when she got pregnant again.

Before abortion: Tense.

During abortion: Pain was severe at times.

After abortion: Weak.

Observations: Retroverted uterus.

Editor's Comment: Her sister also had an abortion at Planned Parenthood during this time period.

Name: Cindy S.

Patient information: Single, member of Assembly of God, no children. Wants children. Took the Pill off and on for one year. Discontinued use and was not using the Pill when she got pregnant.

Before abortion: Overreacted. Tense, nervous, talkative, complaining.

During abortion: Mild pain.

After abortion: Walked, weak.

Observations: Acted twelve years old. Not very responsible for a seventeen-year-old. May be a repeater with birth control attitude. Attitude toward birth control: *Horrible*—says she'll probably quit them but doesn't want any other method. Very immature.

Editor's Comment: Her sister also had two abortions at Planned Parenthood.

Name: Barbara Q.

Patient information: Married, Assembly of God, two children, not sure if she wants more. Used the Pill for six months, now using foam. Was using spermicidal foam when she got pregnant.

Before abortion: Relaxed, some nervousness.

During abortion: Relaxed, quiet, sense of humor. Pain was severe at times.

After abortion: Walked.

Observations:

Name: Barbara Q.

Patient information: Married, Baptist, two children, not sure if she wants more. Used the Pill for six months, then switched to spermicidal foam, then went back to the Pill, then stopped using all contraception. Had a previous abortion (got pregnant while using the foam). Will go back to using the Pill again.

Before abortion:

During abortion:

After abortion:

Observations:

Name: Leigh R.

Patient information: Married, Lutheran, no children, but wants children. Never has used contraception, but intends to use an IUD after the abortion.

Before abortion: Tense, nervous, talkative.

During abortion: Pain was severe at times.

After abortion: Walked.

Observations: No problems noted with decision. Nervous, but did fine.

Name: Betty R.

Patient information: Married, Methodist, two children. Not sure if she wants more children. Used the Pill off and on for five years, but gave it up due to a fibrocyst. Presently using condoms.

Before abortion: Tense, withdrawn, quiet.

During abortion: Mild pain.

After abortion: Walked.

Observations: Betty and her husband were extremely quiet and solemn. Never cracked a smile the whole day. Could not take the Pill, afraid of IUD, and said Diaphragm hurt — so she'll go back to foam and condoms. Said husband wanted vasectomy — sometime. Strange couple.

Name: Elaine R.

Patient information: Single, member of Salvation Army, no children, but does want children. Has never used contraception, but will go on the Pill after the abortion.

Before abortion: Cried, nervous.

During abortion: Mild pain.

After abortion: Walked, talkative.

Observations: Was extremely nervous.

Name: Venus R.

Patient information: Single, Methodist, no children. Wants children. Has never used contraception, but will use the Pill after the abortion.

Before abortion: Tense, nervous, cried.

During abortion: Mild pain.

After abortion: Walked, talkative, sense of humor.

Observations: Venus was very nervous, she started crying when Dr. Leerson first came into the room. I talked with her, Dr. Leerson was very nice to her, and she got control of herself. She did fine during the procedure and came in smiling when she entered T.V. room.

Name: Jovita R.

Patient information: Married, two children. Does not want any more children. Obtained the Pill from Planned Parenthood, used it for only four months. Dropped the Pill due to physical complications. Presently using nothing.

Before abortion: Relaxed, quiet.

During abortion: No pain.

After abortion: Walked.

Observations: Very quiet and dull-witted. Needs that IUD! Procedure very fast and smooth.

Name: Marjory R.

Patient information: Married, Church of Christ, one child. Wants more children. Uses the Pill, but it causes less sexual desire. Missed one Pill last month, but took two the next day. Will stay on the Pill.

Before abortion: Relaxed, talkative.

During abortion: Pain was very severe.

After abortion: Walked, talkative.

Observations:

Name: Maria R.

Patient information: Married, Catholic, one child. Wants more children. Has not used contraceptives, but will use Pill after abortion.

Before abortion: Tense, nervous, quiet.

During abortion: Pain was severe at times.

After abortion: Weak, faint.

Observations: Wouldn't communicate after VPT; withdrew. Extremely nauseated all day. Quiet, non-communicative lady. Problems at home? Briefly mentioned that her daughter had to have surgery as couldn't walk. Wouldn't talk further.

Name: Khadije K.

Patient information: Married, Moslem, two children. Does not want more children. Has never used contraception, but will use the Pill after the abortion.

Before abortion: Quiet.

During abortion: Mild pain.

After abortion: Walked.

Observations: Khadije does not speak any English at all, but her husband does. I explained the procedure, pills, and post-op to him and he relayed them to her. I hope she understands the Pill — at least how to take them. Her husband said they definitely want no more children, but that an operation like the LAP is unheard of by their custom and Moslem religion. I don't think he would admit to himself or to his wife that they were stopping a pregnancy. She was a perfect patient! Left happy.

Name: Jessie R.

Patient information: Single, member of Church of God, no children. Wants children. Used the Pill for three years, presently using foam. Has experienced nausea, dizziness, and cramping.

Before abortion: Relaxed, quiet, sense of humor.

During abortion: Mild pain.

After abortion: Walked.

Observations: Perfect patient! No problems noted.

Name: Debbie R.

Patient information: Single, Baptist, no children, but wants children. Never has used birth control, but will use the Pill after the abortion.

Before abortion: Cried. Tense, withdrawn.

During abortion: Pain was severe at times.

After abortion: Cried. Weak.

Observations: Debbie and her mother had a very good relationship. Her mother told me that Debbie was "seduced" and that she wanted to help her in any way. Debbie was very quiet and melancholy. When I talked to her in private, she said this was her decision and that her mother made her feel very comfortable with it. I'm not sure if she'll continue on the Pill.

Follow Up: Debbie left school yesterday — was nauseous and face was flushed — no fever or bad cramps — fine today. I asked her mother to call us if problems persist.

Name: Rhonda R.

Patient information: Single, Methodist, no children. Not sure if she wants children. Has not used contraception, but will use the Pill after her abortion.

Before abortion: Some nervousness.

During abortion: Quiet. Cried. Mild pain.

After abortion: Weak, vomited.

Observations:

Editor's Comment: Got pregnant again two and a half years later while using the Pill prescribed to her by Planned Parenthood, and had a second abortion at Planned Parenthood.

Name: Rhonda R.

Patient information: Single, Methodist, no children. Not sure if she wants any children. Was prescribed the Pill by Planned Parenthood after her first abortion. Got pregnant again while using the Pill—but will stay on the Pill after the abortion.

Before abortion:

During abortion:

After abortion:

Observations:

Name: Susan R.

Patient information: Married, no children, but wants children. Used the Pill for three years. Presently uses condoms, but not consistently.

Before abortion: Relaxed, realistic, quiet.

During abortion: Mild pain.

After abortion: Walked, weak.

Observations: Susan came in last week to see about a pregnancy test and a VPT. I gave her the information and she asked if it was possible to do it herself. I told her she was risking her life if she did. She seemed very personable today, although she was quiet and was appreciative.

Name: Connie R.

Patient information: Married, Catholic, no living children. Not sure if she wants children.

Before abortion: Tense, nervous, withdrawn, quiet.

During abortion: Pain was severe at times.

After abortion: Walked.

Observations: Very quiet lady. Hard to tell what she was thinking as she did not express herself at all. May have been a language problem? Also, may have been cultural reaction.

Name: Rhonda C.

Patient information: Single, Baptist, no children. Wants children. Has not used contraception, but will get on the Pill after the abortion.

Before abortion:

During abortion:

After abortion:

Observations:

Editor's Comment: Rhonda took the Pill for six months, but did not refill the prescription. She got pregnant again about six months after she stopped the Pill, and had another abortion at Planned Parenthood.

Name: Rhonda C.

Patient information: Single, Baptist, no children. Wants children. Came to Planned Parenthood for an abortion last year. Afterwards, used the Pill for six months. Presently using nothing. Will go back on the Pill after the abortion.

Before abortion: Tense, talkative, sense of humor.

During abortion: Mild pain.

After abortion: Walked.

Observations: Was not too motivated to take Pill (didn't refill last prescription). Neither she nor her mother were very concerned that this was Rhonda's second VPT. Mother appeared overly permissive; offered no guidance. Left in very good spirits.

Name: Cindy R.

Patient information: Single, Baptist, no children. Wants children. Used the Pill for eight months. Has used nothing for last three months.

Before abortion: Tense, talkative, cried.

During abortion: Pain was severe at times.

After abortion: Cried.

Observations: Cried towards end of procedure and after it was over. I talked with her and she said she was just so happy it was over. Arrived in recovery room via wheelchair.

Name: Susan S.

Patient information: Married, Protestant, one child. Not sure if she wants more children. Used the Pill for several years; presently using contraceptive foam; was using foam when she got pregnant. Will use the Pill after the abortion.

Before abortion: Nervous, talkative, realistic, relaxed.

During abortion: No pain.

After abortion: Weak, talkative.

Observations: Had her child naturally and knew how to breathe and concentrate during procedure. It seemed very easy for her and she was a wonderful patient.

Name: Almudena R.

Patient information: Single, Catholic, no children. Unsure if she wants any children. Does not use contraception, but will take the Pill after the abortion.

Before abortion: Tense, nervous, quiet, complaining.

During abortion: Pain was severe at times.

After abortion: Walked.

Observations: Did OK during procedure — very immature. Attitude toward birth control is fair. Does not seem responsible to stay on the Pill.

Name: Mary Beth R.

Patient information: Single, one child, wants more children. Used the Pill off and on for five years (got some prescriptions filled at Planned Parenthood). Presently using foam, but did not use foam when she got pregnant.

Before abortion: Relaxed.

During abortion: Mild pain.

After abortion: Weak. Fainted.

Observations: Came through the procedure fine. Became dizzy and fainted afterwards, but quick recovery. She is an intelligent, responsible person and she will probably take the Pill successfully.

Name: Kallen R.

Patient information: Married, Baptist, no children. Wants children. Has used contraceptive foam for about six months, but did not use foam when she got pregnant.

Before abortion: Tense, nervous, complaining. Overreacted.

During abortion: Mild pain.

After abortion: Walked, talkative.

Observations: Very bad patient. Wouldn't relax at all. Kept pulling back on the table. She was ten to twelve weeks and didn't have much pain but worked herself into a frenzy. Possible repeater.

Name: Karla R.

Patient information: Single, Baptist, no children. Wants children. Does not use contraception, but intends to use the Pill after the abortion.

Before abortion: Tense, nervous, quiet.

During abortion: Pain was severe at times.

After abortion: Walked, talkative.

Observations: To recovery room by wheelchair. No distress noted. Did much better than I anticipated.

Name: Sylvia R.

Patient information: Divorced, Catholic, one child. Wants more children. Used the Pill for one year, but it caused blotches. Has been off the Pill for four years. Presently using nothing.

Before abortion: Tense, nervous, quiet, almost cried.

During abortion: Pain was severe at times.

After abortion: Walked.

Observations: Very retroverted uterus. Nice lady. No problems noted with decision. Reaction seemed appropriate for background.

Name: Thirza R.

Patient information: Married, Catholic, two children. Does not want any more children. Used the Pill for three months, but it caused breakthrough bleeding, nervousness, and nausea. Presently using withdrawal as method of contraception.

Before abortion: Realistic, talkative, nervous.

During abortion: Mild pain.

After abortion: Walked, talkative, sense of humor.

Observations: Nice lady—good husband support. She's very hyper and a worrier. She will probably call several times but I'm sure will be fine. Wants LAP in six weeks and I hope she will follow through. She has trouble remembering things, but not afraid to ask and ask and ask and ask!

Name: Vanessa S.

Patient information: Single, Catholic, no children. Wants children. Uses condoms, was using condom when she got pregnant. Intends to use the Pill after the abortion.

Before abortion: Nervous, realistic, talkative.

During abortion: Pain was severe at times.

After abortion: Walked.

Observations: No problems noted with decision.

Name: Cristina S.

Patient information: Married, Catholic, one child. Wants more children. Does not use contraception, but will use the Pill after the abortion.

Before abortion: Relaxed, realistic, talkative.

During abortion: Mild pain.

After abortion: Walked, talkative.

Observations: Great patient! Smiled all the way through.

Name: Mary S.

Patient information: Separated, one child. Does not want more children. Used the Pill off and on for two years, but the Pill caused nausea. Presently not using contraception, but will take the Pill again after the abortion.

Before abortion: Realistic, talkative, slightly nervous.

During abortion: Mild pain.

After abortion: Walked.

Observations: Excellent patient. No problems noted with decision.

Name: Rose S.

Patient information: Single, Catholic, two children. Wants more children. Has used the Pill for two years, but had missed several when she got pregnant.

Before abortion: Tense, withdrawn, nervous, quiet.

During abortion: Pain was severe at times.

After abortion: Walked, weak.

Observations: Better patient than expected. Just had breast enlargement in April and was still very tender. She seemed a bit emotional before the procedure but seemed fine afterwards. Wants LAP as soon as augmentation is paid. Won't stay on the Pill. Attitude toward birth control: *questionable.*

Name: Carmen S.

Patient information: Single, Catholic, no children, but wants children. Started using the Pill three months ago, after her first abortion. Used the Pill for only one month, got pregnant two months later.

Before abortion: Relaxed, realistic, talkative.

During abortion: None.

After abortion: Walked.

Observations: To recovery room via wheelchair. No distress noted. Very apathetic. Not concerned at all about birth control or repeated abortions (or financial situation). Made wisecracks in VPT room and laughed at inappropriate moments. Unaffected by entire procedure. Attitude toward birth control: *poor.*

Name: Yolanda S.

Patient information: Divorced, one child. Wants more children. Used the Pill for one year; has not used Pill in six years. Pill caused weight gain. Was not using contraception when she got pregnant.

Before abortion:

During abortion:

After abortion:

Observations:

Name: Mary G.

Patient information: Single, Baptist, no children, but does want children. Uses condoms; was using condoms when she got pregnant. Intends to get on the Pill after the abortion.

Before abortion: Nervous, talkative.

During abortion: Pain was severe at times.

After abortion: Weak, faint, nauseated. Walked.

Observations: Recovered quickly. No problems noted.

Name: Laurie S.

Patient information: Single, no children, but wants children. Used the Pill for four months, but developed lump in leg. Presently not using contraception.

Before abortion: Realistic.

During abortion: Mild pain.

After abortion: Walked.

Observations: Did fine. Eight days later: patient called and said she was bleeding and cramping. I told her to come in and see Dr. Wall. Next day: did not answer. Attitude toward birth control: *questionable.*

Name: Patricia S.

Patient information: Single, no children, but does want children. Has used the Pill and a diaphragm, obtained from Planned Parenthood. Presently using the diaphragm; was using the diaphragm when she got pregnant. Will try an IUD after the abortion.

Before abortion: Relaxed, realistic, talkative.

During abortion: Mild pain.

After abortion: Walked, talkative.

Observations: Good patient. Hope IUD works.

Name: Emma S.

Patient information: Separated, Catholic, two children. Not sure if she wants more children. Used the Pill for nine years, but presently is not using contraception.

Before abortion: Realistic, tense, talkative, sense of humor.

During abortion: No pain.

After abortion: Walked.

Observations: Extremely relaxed. Great patient. No problems at all.

Name: Cynthia S.

Patient information: Married, Catholic, four children. Does not want more children. Used the Pill for seven years, but developed breakthrough bleeding. Presently uses condoms.

Before abortion: Relaxed, realistic, talkative.

During abortion: Mild pain.

After abortion: Walked, talkative.

Observations: Very good patient — no problems.

Name: Lorri S.

Patient information: Single, Catholic, no children. Wants children. Has never used contraception, but will take the Pill for one month after the abortion.

Before abortion: Tense, nervous.

During abortion: Pain was severe at times.

After abortion: Walked, talkative.

Observations: Mother and father were both here. Mother cried off and on all day. Think it was hardest on her. Lorri is only sixteen and quite immature. She did much better during VPT than I anticipated. Will take Pill for one month and that is all. Twenty-five days later: patient discontinued the Pill and does not want to use any method of contraception.

Name: Ann S.

Patient information: Single, no children, but does want children. Used the Pill for one year. Presently not using contraception.

Before abortion: Relaxed, realistic, sense of humor.

During abortion: Mild pain.

After abortion: Weak, walked.

Observations: Great patient. Does not trust the Pill or IUD. I think she'll be fine with diaphragm. No problems.

Name: Margaret S.

Patient information: Married, Catholic, three children. Does not want more children. Used the IUD for four years, but it caused increased bleeding. IUD caused inflammation and she had to have an ovary removed. Used the Pill for four years. Presently not using contraception but will use foam and condoms after the abortion.

Before abortion: Tense, nervous, talkative.

During abortion: Mild Pain.

After abortion: Walked.

Observations: To TV room via wheelchair in no apparent distress. Was decided on VPT until husband said "lets have a baby." They talked until 1:00 p.m. and decided on VPT. She was very emotional but has enough maturity to handle the situation.

Name: Jan S.

Patient information: Married, had one child (placed for adoption). Not sure if she wants any children. Used the Pill for five years; discontinued Pill use two months ago.

Before abortion: Relaxed, realistic, talkative.

During abortion: Mild pain.

After abortion: Walked, talkative.

Observations: Very relaxed, good, mature patient! A real change! Seemed to have a good attitude about VPT and birth control.

Name: Cindy F.

Patient information: Single, non-denominational Christian, no children. Wants children. Has never used contraception, but will use the Pill after the abortion.

Before abortion: Realistic, tense, nervous.

During abortion: Pain very severe.

After abortion: Weak.

Observations: Cervix was hard to dilate. Very painful for her.

Name: Helen S.

Patient information: Single, no children. Wants children. Had previous abortion one year ago. Used the Pill for one month after the first abortion. Presently not using contraception.

Before abortion: Nervous, quiet.

During abortion: Mild pain.

After abortion: Walked.

Observations: Seemed very embarrassed by the entire procedure.

Name: Virginia S.

Patient information: Single, Catholic, no children. Wants children. Does not use contraception, but will take the Pill after the abortion.

Before abortion: Overreacted, tense, quiet.

During abortion: Pain was severe at times.

After abortion: Weak.

Observations: Received in recovery room via wheelchair. Very shy and not too bright. Jumped when he put speculum in. He had a hard time dilating the cervix, but she calmed down and did fine, though it was painful.

Name: Bernadine S.

Patient information: Single, no children. Wants children. Uses condoms, but was not using condom when she got pregnant. Will take the Pill after the abortion.

Before abortion: Tense, nervous, quiet.

During abortion: Mild pain.

After abortion: Walked.

Observations: Did fine — no problems. Attitude toward birth control: *afraid of Pill?*

Name: Leslie S.

Patient information: Married, two children. Does not want more children. Was using contraceptive foam when she got pregnant.

Before abortion: Nervous, talkative, realistic.

During abortion: Mild pain.

After abortion: Walked, talkative, sense of humor, weak.

Observations: Very nice woman! Seemed to be comfortable with her decision.

Editor's Comment: Used the Pill for almost a year, then got pregnant again while still on the Pill and had her second abortion at Planned Parenthood.

Name: Alice Q.

Patient information: Married, Catholic, two children. Does not want any more children. Used Pill off and on for eight years, presently using nothing. Intends to use the Pill again after the abortion.

Before abortion: Nervous, talkative.

During abortion: Mild pain.

After abortion: Walked.

Observations: No problems noted with decision. Nice lady.

Name: Mary H.

Patient information: Single, Catholic, no children, but does want children. Does not use contraception, but will take the Pill after the abortion.

Before abortion:

During abortion:

After abortion:

Observations: Seemed disinterested in all information given. She may not stay on the Pill since her interest in birth control and VPT was low! Attitude toward birth control: *only fair.*

Name: Donna J.

Patient information: Single, Episcopal, no children. Does not want any children. Used the Pill for two years, but had several physical problems. Presently not using contraception. Will not consider any method of contraception after the abortion.

Before abortion: Relaxed, realistic, talkative.

During abortion: Mild pain.

After abortion: Walked, talkative, sense of humor.

Observations: Good patient—good VPT attitude. Attitude toward birth control: *not a Pill taker*—too many problems but will check with her private medical doctor—would not consider other methods.

Name: Denise S.

Patient information: Married, Jewish, no children. Wants children. Received birth control from Planned Parenthood three years ago. Used the Pill but discontinued it. Will use the Pill after the abortion.

Before abortion: Relaxed.

During abortion: Mild pain. Some difficulty dilating cervix. Had to use smaller suction tube.

After abortion: Walked.

Observations: Excellent patient. Good support from husband.

Name: Mary P.

Patient information: Single, Baptist, no children—and doesn't want any. Has never used contraception, but will use the Pill after the abortion.

Before abortion: Nervous, realistic.

During abortion: Very severe pain.

After abortion: Weak, was faint and nauseous.

Observations: Good patient despite her cramps, weakness, etc. Light headed. Firm in decision. No problems noted. Nice girl.

Name: Jane P.

Patient information: Divorced, Unity Church member, no children. Wants children. Used the Pill off and on for four years, but presently uses nothing. Will use the Pill again after the abortion.

Before abortion: Nervous, talkative, realistic.

During abortion: Pain was severe at times.

After abortion: Weak, faint, walked.

Observations: Good patient — mature attitude. No problems expected.

Name: Stephaney P.

Patient information: Married, Baptist, has one child and does want more children. Was a Pill user, but discontinued use. Was using spermicidal foam when she got pregnant. Intends to go back to the Pill after the abortion.

Before abortion: Realistic, relaxed.

During abortion: Mild pain.

After abortion: Walked, sense of humor.

Observations: Good patient! No problems noted with the decision. Nice lady.

Name: Denise D.

Patient information: Married, no children, but wants children. Has used the Pill and spermicides, but was using nothing when she got pregnant. Intends to use the Pill after the abortion.

Before abortion: Relaxed.

During abortion: Mild pain. Some difficulty dilating cervix—had to use smaller cannulas.

After abortion: Relieved, happy.

Observations: Excellent patient—good support from husband.

Name: Patty P.

Patient information: Single, no children, but wants children. Has used the Pill and diaphragm—was using diaphragm when she got pregnant. Intends to use the Pill after the abortion.

Before abortion: Tense, nervous, talkative.

During abortion: Pain was severe at times.

After abortion: Weak, dry heaved, walked.

Observations: Pain hard for her—decision was firm.

Name: Elaine P.

Patient information: Married, one child, wants more children. Former Pill user, was using diaphragm when she got pregnant. Intends to go back to the Pill after the abortion.

Before abortion: Relaxed, realistic, talkative, sense of humor.

During abortion: No pain.

After abortion: Walked, talkative.

Observations: Was an excellent patient. Used the same breathing techniques she used during natural childbirth and she didn't budge.

Name: Mary Dolores A.

Patient information: Married, Catholic, no children, but wants children. Condom user, was using condoms when she got pregnant. Intends to get on the Pill after the abortion.

Before abortion: Tense, talkative, nervous, overreacted.

During abortion: Pain was severe at times. Cramped hard—not used to cramping. Wiggled a lot. Dr. was relatively patient with her.

After abortion: Walked, was relieved.

Observations: Decision—no problems noted. Support from husband. Reaction seemed normal for background.

Name: Leticia P.

Patient information: Single, no children, but wants children. In her words: "Well, I am not married and sixteen years of age. I want to finish school. I feel I'm doing the right thing. But don't know. . . ." Never has used birth control, but intends to get on the Pill after the abortion.

Before abortion: Quiet.

During abortion: Mild pain.

After abortion: Walked, talkative, relieved, quiet.

Observations: Dull senses.

Name: Shirley Jo P.

Patient information: Married, Catholic, no children, but wants children. Former Pill user, now usually uses condoms. Stopped using Pill three months ago due to physical complications (sluggishness, bloating). Believes that she will have a "sense of relief and sadness" after the abortion.

Before abortion: Tense, realistic, talkative.

During abortion: Pain was severe at times.

After abortion: Walked, talkative, sense of humor.

Observations: Darling patient — trying so hard to be a good patient. Her legs stuck straight out from exam on. Seemed very sure of her decision and was going back on Pill for sure.

Name: Mattie P.

Patient information: Single, Methodist, one child. Does not want more children. Used the Pill for eight years. The Pill made her nauseous. Presently not using contraception, but intends to have an IUD inserted after the abortion.

Before abortion: Tense, quiet, realistic.

During abortion: Mild pain.

After abortion: Walked, talkative.

Observations: A very quiet woman. The procedure was fairly easy for her. I'm glad she got an IUD because I doubt she would be a very good Pill taker. She's taking diet pills.

Name: Parminder S.

Patient information: Married, no children, but does want children. Uses foam and condoms. Intends to use an IUD after the abortion.

Before abortion: Cried. Tense, talkative, nervous. Overreacted.

During abortion: Pain was severe at times.

After abortion: Walked, talkative.

Observations: To recovery room via wheelchair in no apparent distress. I can't believe she's a doctor. On 11/xx/xx: Mr. Sams called. His wife has continued to bleed since VPT on 9/xx/xx. She had returned for her check-up and was told all was fine. From birth control chart—negative UCG, uterus enlarged but firm, 10/xx/xx. In the last several days the bleeding has worsened. Mr. Sams had already spoken with Dr. Fredricks and had made a tentative appointment for his wife this P.M. I spoke with the nurse practitioner, who had stated she would also be willing to examine Parminder, with the understanding if there was a problem, she would have to refer Parminder on to Dr. Fredricks or to a hospital E.R. Mr. Sams would try to bring his wife to PPH today as our location was more convenient for them. 11:30: Mr. Sams called again. His wife's bleeding had worsened, and they were to see Dr. Fredricks at 2:30. I asked that he call me and let me know what happened. 11/12/76: Uterus was normal size. He spoke with her this date and bleeding had slacked off slightly— K. Watson. Parminder has not been taking pills—K. Watson 11/15/76: Parminder was seen by Dr. Fredricks.

Name: Sylvia S.

Patient information: Single, no children, wants children. Uses condoms; was using condoms when she got pregnant.

Before abortion: Sense of humor, talkative, nervous.

During abortion: Pain was very severe.

After abortion: Fainted, vomited, weak.

Observations: Sylvia cooperated fully but had a very difficult time. Was weak and couldn't sit up for ten minutes after the procedure. Pain continued a long time. Received in recovery room via wheelchair. Very nauseous. Left happy.

Birth Control and Abortion

Even if birth control methods were reliable, that is not to say that birth control could ever really prevent unintended pregnancies and abortions, because there are a lot of people who cannot or will not voluntarily use birth control consistently over realistically long-term periods, as the preceding ninety-two abortion files obtained from PPHSET clearly show.

Although 75% of these women were past or current contraceptors, even *after* their abortions, many of the women still did not hold good attitudes toward using birth control: the attitude of 20% was considered "poor," "terrible," "questionable," "horrible," "very questionable," or worse, and the attitudes of another 15% were considered only fair (or an equivalent response connoting some hesitancy or reservation). *Only 37% had attitudes toward birth control that were rated as "good" or "okay" or better.*

It is quite likely that many of the poor attitudes toward birth control stemmed more from actual experience than from callousness or irresponsibility. After all, 75% of the abortions were performed on women who were current or past birth control users, and at least 13% had previously been PPHSET customers.

These women's bad attitudes toward birth control evolved as much from the plethora of physical problems associated with the different methods as from uncaring or unrealistic personal outlooks.

But if these ninety-two abortion files demonstrate that dispensing birth control is not the solution to preventing unintended pregnancy and abortion, they also reveal the true cause of abortion: family planning. *Over 80% of the abortions were performed on women who said they wanted more children,*[2] *just not right now.*

In addition, one-third of the women who had the abortions were married, and only 29% of these women said they did not want any more children. Of the 67% who were unmarried, only 14% said they did not want more children.

Seventy-five percent of the women had used or were using birth control, and 80% of them wanted more children, and yet *all* of them had abortions? Clearly, the reason these ninety-two women had abortions was not that they failed to use family planning: The ninety-two abortions were the direct result of family planning.

---

2. Sixty-seven percent who definitely wanted more and 13% who "maybe" wanted more.

Aborting a child is the ultimate act of family planning. To these women, the value of a child was dependent upon how conveniently timed his arrival would be: A child held no intrinsic value except to enrich the life of his mother by a correctly timed birth.

Family Planning and the Value of Children

It is the acceptance and internalization of the dogma of family planning that causes unplanned pregnancies, unwanted children, and abortion. Without acceptance of family planning, the concepts of unintended pregnancy, unwanted child, and abortion simply do not exist. It is acceptance of the belief that children should be wanted, or should be born only with the permission of the parents, and only upon their timetable, which gives meaning to "unplanned pregnancy," " unintended pregnancy," and "unwanted child."

To understand what I'm saying, you have to envision a world in which family planning simply does not exist. In this world, children are accepted as gifts from God, creations with intrinsic worth. Children have an intrinsic worth because they are made in the image of God.

The concept of "unplanned pregnancies" has no meaning if you reject the belief that pregnancies should be planned. The concept of "unwanted children" has no meaning if you reject the notion that children must be wanted. The concept of "unintended pregnancy" has no meaning if you reject the belief that all pregnancies ought to be intentional.

The point is this: "Unwanted children" and "unplanned pregnancies" are inherent to the very definition of family planning. By definition, family planning values *planned* pregnancies, *wanted* children, *intended* conceptions, and by definition, these planned pregnancies, wanted children, and intended conceptions are good and valuable. And, conversely, since planned pregnancies are good and valuable, *un*planned pregnancies are bad and valueless. Since wanted children are good and valuable and desirable, *un*wanted children are bad and valueless and undesirable.

But it is important to see that these concepts of wantedness and planning are merely one arbitrary way of looking at pregnancy. If you reject the importance or validity of family planning, you reject the importance or validity of analyzing a pregnancy in terms of whether it was planned.

Planned Parenthood is always claiming that family planning strengthens families, and that its systematic extermination of unwanted children increases the value and wantedness of the children who are allowed to continue living. But family planning devalues children.

Family planning has devalued children because it has made them expendable. Family planning has transformed children, both born and unborn, from human beings with intrinsic worth into life enrichment units whose value and continued existence are subject solely to the whims of their parents. Children serve no legitimate purpose other than to enrich the lives of their parents, or to contribute to society as a whole (which is a polite way of saying that the advocates of family planning do not place a very high value on a wanted child who is the offspring of a black unmarried welfare recipient). Family planning has redefined children as the property of their parents (especially of their mothers). In family planning, parents own their children and they can buy and sell them (as in surrogate mother cases) or kill them if they choose to do so (as in abortion and the starvation of Baby Doe) — no questions asked.

Family planning defines being unwanted as a death penalty crime. Under family planning, the unwanted child is punished for the faults of his parents: No infant ever asked to be unwanted. If a child is unwanted, it's certainly not the child's fault. If a baby's parents don't want him, it's the parents who have the defect, a real lack of love and selflessness. But family planning legitimizes the hardheartedness of parents who do not "want" their children, and it allows the most self-centered and unloving of parents to exercise the power of life and death over their innocent, helpless children.

The root cause of abortion, then, is clearly family planning, not a failure to use contraception.[3] If you reject family planning,

---

3. Other authors have documented the role of family planning in increasing the incidence of abortion. In *Abortion and the Politics of Motherhood* (Berkeley: University of California, 1984), Kristin Luker points to the birth control pill as one of the factors in influencing the increased demand for abortion during the 1960s: "perhaps the pill played a more indirect role in encouraging support for abortion. Mariano Requena has found that in Latin America the introduction of more effective contraception led to an increase in the abortion rate. He argues that after couples have made a commitment to lower fertility, they are less willing to tolerate mistakes when they occur."

you reject all the philosophical justifications for abortion. Abortion is not the inevitable result of a failure to use family planning; quite the contrary, abortion is the inevitable result of acceptance of the family planning mentality.

Societal Effects of Family Planning

Family planning was originally sold as being more healthful because it allowed mothers to space the births of their children, allowing their bodies and spirits a longer rest period between births.

It is astounding, then, to discover that modern family planning has in fact yielded no measurable effect on the birth spacing of American women.[4]

MEDIAN INTERVAL BETWEEN BIRTHS

Race and Interval	Year of Birth of Child	
White	**1965-1969**	**1930-1934**
Median interval in months from:		
— First marriage of mother to birth of first child	15.5	20.3
— Birth of first child to birth of second child	29.3	32.2
— Birth of second child to birth of third child	33.1	31.8
— Birth of third child to birth of fourth child	35.0	33.1
Total months of spacing	112.9	117.49
Negro	**1960-1964**	**1940-1944**
Median interval in months from:		
— First marriage of mother to birth of first child	9.0	10.7
— Birth of first child to birth of second child	23.3	27.3
— Birth of second child to birth of third child	23.8	24.1
— Birth of third child to birth of fourth child	22.1	24.0
Total months of spacing	78.2	86.1

---

4. *Source:* U.S. Bureau of the Census, *Historical Statistics of the United States, Colonial Times to 1970, part 1*, (Washington, D.C., 1975), p. 55. Data shown represent the widest available time intervals.

As family planning has been internalized by Americans over the last fifty to sixty years, and especially since the introduction of the Pill in the very early 1960s, we have not witnessed the considerable health benefits we expected; rather tens of thousands of women have been harmed by legal and illegal abortions, chemical contraceptives, and venereal disease.

In short, family planning has not delivered on any of its promises: It has not enhanced the health of American women by longer birth spacing (the spacings have *decreased* as family planning has become more widespread);[5] unintended pregnancies have soared; teen pregnancies have soared; illegitimate births have soared; venereal diseases have become near-epidemic; child abuse has soared; female poverty and the number of single parent families have soared; and tens of millions of children have been aborted. All the things that family planning was supposed to cure, it has significantly worsened.

The near-universal acceptance of family planning and birth control has not restructured the composition or birth spacing of the American family nearly so much as it has reshaped the attitudes of Americans toward families and children.

Since advocates of family planning and birth control focus on sexual consequences rather than sexual behaviors, they see nothing wrong with intercourse outside of marriage. They unfailingly define illegitimate births as a failure to use birth control, a *technical* failure, rather than as a failure to refrain from improper sexual relations, a *moral* failure.

Family planning has fueled the growth of sexual relations outside of marriage.

Indeed, there is much statistical evidence that acceptance of birth control and family planning have loosened the cultural barriers to premarital and extramarital sex. This explosion of

5. Although birth spacings have decreased, total fertility has declined, primarily due to the fact that so many married couples now resort to surgical sterilization. More than 30% of married women aged thirty-five to forty-four have been surgically sterilized, as have more than 20% of husbands of women aged thirty-five to forty-four. See, for instance, National Center for Health Statistics, W. D. Mosher and C. A. Bachrach: Contraceptive Use, United States, 1982, *Vital and Health Statistics*, series 23, no. 12. DHHS pub. no. (PHS)86-1988. Public Health Service. (Washington, D.C.: U.S. Government Printing Office, September 1986), table 5.

sex outside of marriage has put tremendous strains upon birth control, necessitating that contraceptive methods work flawlessly for increasingly protracted time periods.

For instance, of women who married between 1960 and 1964, only 9.2% had been sexually active for 36 months or longer, including 2.9% who were sexually active for 60 months or longer before marriage. But for women who married between 1975 and 1979, the comparable figures were 40.4% and 23.4%, respectively.[6] *Thus, in order to avoid a rise in the rate of pregnancy for unmarried women, birth control would have had to work flawlessly for at least three years for almost three times as many women, and for at least five years for eight times as many women!*

STRAINS ON BIRTH CONTROL: TIMING OF MARRIAGE RELATIVE TO FIRST SEXUAL INTERCOURSE FOR EVER-MARRIED WOMEN: 1982 (WOMEN AGED 15-44 ONLY)

Year of First Marriage	Percent Distribution Months Between First Intercourse and Marriage					
	Same Month	< 6	6-11	12-35	36-59	60 or >
1960-1964	44.1	17.1	8.6	20.9	6.3	2.9
1975-1979	20.6	6.6	7.2	25.1	17.0	23.4

The statistics for unmarried cohabitation similarly highlight how loosened sexual mores have strained birth control.[7] For instance, in 1970 there were 523,000 unmarried couples, of which 196,000 had children under fifteen. By 1985, these figures had risen to 1,983,000 unmarried couples, including 603,000 with children under fifteen. Virtually all of this increase came in couples under forty-four years of age, that is, of childbearing age. The number of cohabiting couples under age twenty-five increased 772%, while the number of cohabiting couples aged twenty-five to forty-four rose 1,167%. Since cohabiting couples have lower desires for children, this tremendous increase has put a significant strain on birth control, has seriously distorted the statistics on illegitimate births, and has led to hundreds of thousands of abortions.

---

6. *Statistical Abstract of the United States: 1987,* no. 98, p. 66.
7. *Statistical Abstract of the United States, 1987,* no. 54, p. 42.

The introduction of the Pill, the legalization of abortion, and the proliferation of Planned Parenthood-style sex indoctrination classes have helped to foster a false perception that sex outside of marriage is both acceptable and safe. Americans have been greatly deceived into a false belief that birth control effectively prevents pregnancies. But it is clear that birth control does not prevent pregnancies, it only makes them somewhat less likely compared to non-contracepted intercourse. The tremendous increase in the average length of premarital sexual activity, and the tremendous rise in unmarried cohabitation, have made the surge in "unintended" pregnancies inevitable — inevitable because over time, most people who use birth control will become unintentionally pregnant. And of these, most will resort to abortion as their backup method of "birth control."

Summary

We will not be able to vanquish abortion by means of family planning, because abortion is really the logical conclusion of family planning; abortion is really just one more method of "birth control" and just one more tool in family planning's war on inconveniently timed children.

All of the abortions detailed in the preceding 92 records were crimes of convenience. There were no rape cases, no incestuous conceptions, no unmarried welfare mothers with 12 children, no diagnoses of fetal deformity, no women who had been denied access to affordable contraceptive services, no 11-year-old honor students, no mothers in physiological danger due to pregnancy.

Before performing the abortions, Planned Parenthood asked each woman "How do you think you will feel after the termination?" Their responses demonstrated the callous and often flippant reasons why these women resorted to abortion (not all responded):

- I would rather have this done. I couldn't accept the responsibility of a child yet.
- Relief.
- Happy & content with my two children I have.
- It was best for me.
- Fine.
- Relieved; glad it's over. Do not want children now.

- Relaxed.
- O.K.
- I think it's the best thing I could do.
- Alright. I don't feel a child right now would be good for me.
- A little sad but relieved.
- Relieved.
- Great.
- I don't know since I've never experienced this before.
- N.A.
- Probably better than I do now.
- Better.
- Relieved.
- I don't think it will bother me a great deal.
- Fine.
- Not really wanted it. But was the best for right now.
- Different.
- Relieved.
- Scared.
- As if it never happened.
- Relieved.
- I hope I'll feel better.
- Relieved.
- I'll feel like this was the best thing I could have done.
- Relieved.
- Okay.
- I don't believe it will affect me that much.
- Relieved.
- That is hard to say, as I've never experienced this before.
- We made the right decision for this particular time in our life.
- That it was the right decision for me.
- Good.
- No comments.
- Well, I am not married and 16 years of age, I want to finish school. I feel I'm doing the right thing. But don't know [?????].
- The same.
- Relief.
- Relief.
- Don't know.
- I think I will be able to live the same life.
- Terrible.

- I am not sure.
- ?
- Great. Will take pill religiously.
- Fine.
- ?
- Normal.
- OK.
- Won't know till after its over.
- I don't know.
- Tranquila.
- I don't know, but I'll be glad it's over with.
- Better.
- Crampy.
- Fine.
- Fine, maybe a little weak.
- No muy contenta.
- I don't know—I really don't want to think about it.
- Sense of relief and sadness.
- That at this time in my life its for the best.
- Better.
- Better!
- Tranquilla mejor.
- Don't know.

Many people naively cling to the belief that abortion would stop if people—mothers, doctors, abortuary staff, pastors, husbands, boyfriends—could just be given enough information to understand that a fetus is a baby, and a baby is a person, and that abortion is murder. Sadly, this belief is false (and probably never was true).

The people who cut up little babies in their mothers' tummies know what they are doing. Mothers pregnant with kicking children know what they are doing when they pay the doctor to kill them.

The reason people get abortions is not ignorance, it is selfishness. The problem is not that abortionists, abortuary staff, and parents do not know that abortion is murder: the problem is that we have reached a point in America where we have decided that certain kinds of murder are excusable or justifiable or necessary or beneficial. It is no longer sufficient to say that abortion is murder; we must also assert that God said, "Thou shalt not kill."

PART TWO

SOLUTIONS

SEVEN

CHOOSING A VISION

The battle against Planned Parenthood is not a battle over which weapons to employ in the fight against teen pregnancy. Planned Parenthood's goal is not the abolition of teen pregnancy; teen pregnancy is merely the rationale and excuse for Planned Parenthood's all out war against the last vestiges of Christian morality and culture in America.

The war against Planned Parenthood is a war of competing worldviews, of competing visions for the future.

Planned Parenthood's vision of the future is a socialist and Swedenized America in which American society, government, and youth have been liberated from the "divisive" influence of traditional Christianity and the moral code that has undergirded Western Civilization from the beginning.

Although it is a near-universal finding of studies on teen promiscuity that frequent attendance at religious services is the best indicator of below-average rates of promiscuity, the Planned Parenthood vision of the future is one in that religion has been banished to irrelevance.

Planned Parenthood does not call for greater parental or church efforts to encourage religious belief and practice; in fact, Planned Parenthood calls for the expunging of religion from any role in sex education, and from any role in formulating or influencing governmental policy.[1]

Planned Parenthood's frightening vision is a logical extension of the personal beliefs of the pro-choice activists that it comprises. In her study, *Abortion and the Politics of Motherhood*, Kristin Luker makes this point very succinctly:

---

1. See for example, Elise F. Jones, et al., "Teen Pregnancy in Developed Countries: Determinants and Policy Implications," *Family Planning Perspectives*, 17:2 (New York: Alan Guttmacher Institute, March/April, 1985).

Perhaps the single most dramatic difference between the two groups [pro-life and pro-choice activists], however, is in the role that religion plays in their lives. Almost three-quarters of the pro-choice people interviewed said that formal religion was either unimportant or completely irrelevant to them, and their attitudes are correlated with behavior: only 25 percent of the pro-choice women said they *ever* attend church, and most of these said they do so only occasionally. Among pro-life people, by contrast, 69 percent said religion was important in their lives, and an additional 22 percent said that it was very important. For pro-life women, too, these attitudes are correlated with behavior: half of those pro-life women interviewed said they attend church regularly once a week, and another 13 percent said they do so even more often. Whereas 80 percent of the pro-choice people never attend church, only 2 percent of pro-life advocates never do so.[2]

The vision doesn't end with the banishment of Christianity. Planned Parenthood wants to liberate our children from *all* influences — parental, religious, educational, and social — that discourage sexual activity outside the context of faithful monogamous marriage. Planned Parenthood acknowledges the role of sex-saturated media in exacerbating teen promiscuity, yet it does not call for *less* sex on the airwaves, but for *more*. It wants fornication presented as responsible (i.e., contracepted) sex. It insists that America must abandon teens to a world of amorality in which "pregnancy, rather than adolescent sexual activity itself, is identified as the major problem."[3]

We are engaged in a battle for the minds and souls of our children, and for the future of our nation. Planned Parenthood understands this battle in ways that its opposition does not, that is why Planned Parenthood is continually calling for compulsory K-12 Planned Parenthood-style sex indoctrination, for sex education that is based on situational ethics rather than morality, and for defining consequences, rather than behaviors, as problematic.

Planned Parenthood's America is a militantly secular, sex-saturated America, and it knows how it wants to get us there:

2. Kristin Luker, *Abortion and the Politics of Motherhood* (Berkeley: University of California, 1984), p. 196-197.
3. Elise F. Jones, et al., p. 61.

. . . universal education in sexuality and contraception; development of special clinics — closely associated with the schools — where young people receive contraceptive services and counseling; free, widely available and confidential contraception and abortion services; widespread advertising of contraceptives in all media; frank treatment of sex; and availability of condoms from a variety of sources.[4]

It must be understood that Planned Parenthood's vision of the future is a vision of national ruin: All of the Western European nations that have embraced Planned Parenthood's vision are dying nations, culturally and demographically. All of them have below-replacement-level birthrates: They are literally contracepting and aborting themselves into oblivion. Sweden, a model of a sex-saturated and secular society that has abandoned God and religion and traditional Western moral standards, has a birthrate more than 40% below the replacement level. Sweden is dying fast.

Planned Parenthood's vision is one of failure: The failure of parents to raise their children correctly, the failure of churches to impart grace and vision to disenchanted teens, the failure of teens to resist peer pressure, the failure of American society to protect teens from pornographic media onslaughts, the failure of schools to provide any encouragement to chastity. To embrace Planned Parenthood's vision is to admit defeat and to call for more failure, to reverse moral failure by reversing morality.

Unfortunately, many Americans, including many Christians, have accepted Planned Parenthood's vision of failure. The common perception is that moral approaches to teen pregnancy have been rendered obsolete by the peer pressure and social pressure that bombard teens.[5]

---

4. Ibid.
5. It should be noted that research seems to show that the adverse influence of the media on teen sexual behavior is indirect. What teens see and hear on television and in the movies has less negative effect than how teens perceive their peers' judgments of what they have seen and heard. Thus, peer pressure acts as a buffer zone between media content and teen sexual behavior, and this peer pressure can either invalidate or intensify media influence. For instance Planned Parenthood's 1986 teen sex poll, found that only 3% of American teens cited "influenced by media" as a reason why teens don't delay having sex; on the other hand, 90% cited peer pressure or a variant thereof as a rea-

It is imperative that we fully reject this vision of failure. The alternative to too much peer pressure should be less peer pressure, not more. The alternative to too much sex on television should be less sex on TV, not more. The alternative to moral failure should be moral success, not more failure. The alternative to too little church teaching on the proper role of sex should be more church teaching on sex, not less.

This vision of failure has sapped American moral vision for too long. It was this same vision of failure that led America to buy into the population explosion hysteria of the 1970s: We saw the solution to distribution-caused food shortages as less people rather than better food distribution.

It is this same vision of moral failure that leads many Americans to embrace oppressive right-wing dictatorships because they believe that the only possible alternative to a bad government is a worse one (e.g., a communist government). The Philippines is an example of the error of this vision. The alternative to a bad Marcos regime was not communism, as we had been told; rather, it was a better and more democratic and fairer government. And so it is with South Africa. The alternative to a cruel and racist government in South Africa is not a communist government, but a less cruel and racist republican government.

Those who hold to the vision of failure too long risk seeing their worst prophecies fulfilled. By supporting the wicked Marcos regime for too long, the United States almost made a communist takeover inevitable by giving the communists sufficient just cause for inciting rebellion.

So it is with teen promiscuity. If we do not soon make a clean break with the pervasive vision of failure that Planned Parenthood promotes, we risk giving Planned Parenthood sufficient rationale for demanding the implementation of more coercive anti-natal

---

son why teens don't delay having sex (*American Teens Speak*, p. 24). Watching X-rated movies does not lead *directly* to first-time teen sexual intercourse; however, teen peer group judgments that X-rated movies depict behavior that is fun, desirable, and normal for teens might become the necessary aggravant to provoke teen first-time sexual intercourse. The conclusion is that we can start solving teen premarital pregnancy without having to clean up the media environment first, if we will begin to reshape teen peer group attitudes toward promiscuity and pornography.

programs. If parents, schools, media, and churches continue to promote only failure and a "not-my-problem" attitude toward premarital sexual behavior, then inevitably Planned Parenthood's totalitarian, governmental, amoral approach will be viewed as reasonable and necessary.

America stands at a crossroads. We can choose the way of life for ourselves, our families, our children, and our nation, or we can allow Planned Parenthood to lead us into the Brave New World of sexual liberation, and spiritual, national, and cultural death.

The choice is ours, and it's a life or death decision.

If we are to have a vision of life, a vision of success for our children, we are first going to have to return to a love of children. We are going to have to return to a high regard for children, not as life enrichment units but as creations made in the image of God, precious gifts with eternal souls, wonderful blessings whose development and maturation are to be zealously guarded from hellish ensnarements.

We need to return to a holistic and comprehensive view of children that acknowledges them as possessing minds and bodies and souls and spirits. We must once again be concerned that our children choose life, rather than just hoping that if they choose death they somehow avoid the worst consequences. We must emphatically concern ourselves with our children's behavior rather than merely with the consequences of their behavior.

Because we no longer care about our children's souls, we express deep concern about illegitimate births, but little or no concern about premarital promiscuity. This concern is selfish: We care more about avoiding welfare babies than we do about the spiritual and emotional health of the fornicator. When we value children in the whole sense we will see premarital promiscuity as a spiritual and emotional tragedy rather than as some inevitable experience of modern maturation.

No one who truly values children as human beings made in the image of God, as creations with an immortal soul, can turn his back upon those children and abandon them to be seduced and defiled by the flood of filth that bombards us daily. We must stand up and fight for our children, for their innocence, and for their future. In the time of greatest temptation, they need our hearts and our help, not 28-day Pill packets.

Teens need information and exhortation and discipleship and guidance and virtuous examples to imitate. They don't need adults to pretend that there are no rules, that behaviors are irrelevant, or that there are no wrong behaviors, only wrong consequences. We require them to learn the rules of the road and to get a license before they can drive a car, but we pretend that there are no rules of sexual conduct and that no marriage license is needed; then we act shocked and dismayed when we find out that they have had a sexual collision where a sperm crashed into an egg and made a baby.

The solution to America's premarital pregnancy crisis is not to Swedenize America by abandoning our teens to secular sexual hedonism, abject moral failure, and national extinction. The solution to America's premarital pregnancy crisis is *faith* and *works*: faith that success can succeed, and hard work by parents and churches and schools and teens to reduce peer pressure, shield teens from social pressure, and develop environments that promote chastity and self-control as a rewarding lifestyle of health and true freedom.

Will it work? Of course it will work. It worked for hundreds of years (before 1960, when we became smarter than history), and it's working even now. The reason poor people's premarital pregnancy rates are far higher than the rest of America's is that very poor people have no vision of success. They believe themselves doomed to poverty and failure and illegitimacy and broken marriages and illiteracy. "Where there is no vision, the people perish."

Will it work? It's already working. Teens who frequently attend religious services are far less promiscuous than any other group of teens. Teens whose parents have given them a vision for marital success and for educational success are less likely to engage in premarital intercourse.

The real question is not "will it work?" but, "will *we* work?" Will we?

Will we go to work as parents and pastors and school teachers and elected officials to make America a better place to live for children and families? Will we stand up for what is good and right and fight for our children? Will we protect them from a wicked adult society hellbent upon stealing their innocence, defiling their purity, and darkening their vision?

Will we care enough as parents to zealously guard the environment our children live in, to protect them from psychological and spiritual molestation? Will we transmit to our children a vision of success, a vision of true freedom and happiness that comes from self-control and life-oriented thinking in all areas of life? Will we raise our children with positive reasons to say no to drugs, no to premarital sex, no to drunkenness, no to debauchery and hedonism, no to pornography, and yes to virginity, yes to abstinence, yes to purity and self-control?

Teaching our children to "just say no" is not enough. Laws alone won't save our nation, our souls, or our children. It is not enough to just tell our children what *not* to do. Neither children nor adults respond well to sterile, negative admonitions to "touch not, taste not, handle not." Children must receive the grace of our vision and encouragement if they are to be expected to stay within the boundaries of life-affirming behaviors.

Merely laying down the law only makes people want to do what's prohibited. What our children need is not repressive approaches to sex that treat sex as a completely isolated, severable facet of life or as an unmentionable, taboo subject.

Neither the Planned Parenthood "sex-is-right-if-it's-right-for-you" approach nor the "sex-does-not-exist-and-if-it-does-don't-do-it-until-you're-married" approach to sex are realistic, moral, or life affirming. Both approaches are failures, and both rob teens of a clear vision of success.

Parents and churches must become sex educators, not in the technical, pedagogical sense so much as in the discipleship sense. Parents and churches must quit pretending that they have less influence over our children than do the television and *Cosmopolitan* magazine. If the television set has more influence over your children than you do, then perhaps it's time you talked to your children more than Tom Selleck and Joan Collins do.

Parents and churches must forsake any latent distaste for sex education and become active sex educators in the fullest sense. Sex education is not inherently immoral. Sure, there are immoral sex education programs, *à la* Planned Parenthood, but that doesn't render all sex education evil. If we don't transmit information and values to our children about sex, someone else will: Planned Parenthood, Sheena Easton, Prince, Eleanor Smeal, Johnny Rotten, and Bill Murray.

Churches should quit pretending that the Bible is silent about sex education. Nothing could be further from the truth. It is the Bible that gives us the clear, consistent vision of the purpose of sex, the right and wrong uses of sex, the freedoms arising from premarital sexual self-control, the beauty of sex within marriage (ever read the Song of Solomon? Ever read it *in church*?), the disastrous consequences of sex outside of marriage, the miraculous nature of procreation, the blessedness and desirability of children and families, the intense, almost mystical, one-flesh bonding of marriage, the wrath of God on sexual perversion, and the proper respect that we should have for one another's bodies and souls.

Sex and procreation are among the most fundamental of all issues of human life, and yet most churches completely ignore discussion of sex and procreation. A truly balanced church will teach from the Song of Solomon as well as from the Epistle to Titus, and a truly balanced church will not feel compelled to pretend that the Song of Solomon is merely spiritual allegory.

Sex education in churches should encourage parent-child communication and should clearly delineate the two pathways of sexual behavior: life and death.[6] Children must be given a clear vision of the two pathways and their consequences, and they must be encouraged and instructed to choose the pathway of life, the lifestyle of chastity and self-control.

Contrary to popular belief, it is not unconstitutional for schools to teach morality. Morality, like religion, is an inescapable concept. Atheism is not the absence of religion; it is the hatred of God. It is not possible to avoid teaching some code of morality. If we teach students that sex is acceptable only within marriage, that is a moral position. If we teach that sex is acceptable outside of marriage, that is also a moral (or immoral) position. The question, then, is not whether schools should teach morality, but which morality schools should teach.

It is far too late for our schools to still be teaching amoral or immoral Planned Parenthood-style sex and contraceptive educa-

---

6. An excellent sex education curriculum for churches is available from Life Advocates in Houston, Texas. Write Life Advocates, One West Loop South, Suite 811, Houston, Texas 77027, and ask for *Choices and Consequences: God's Design for Sexuality.*

tion. If nothing else, AIDS and herpes and genital warts have exposed the "give-'em-birth-control" approach to sex education as the unrealistic failure that it is.

Our schools must quit pretending that premarital teen sexual intercourse is the result of a lack of sexual knowledge, or that premarital teen pregnancy can be effectively reduced by sitting in a class for one hour a day talking about sex. Our schools must institute positive measures to reduce the atmosphere of peer pressure that is the primary aggravator of premarital teen promiscuity.

Schools should implement a holistic, environmental, and peer pressure approach to reducing premarital teen promiscuity, rather than relying on the present isolated approach that regards sex education as another course. Schools should use posters, films, plays, public speakers, and classrooms to provide encouragement to teens' majority lifestyles of chastity, to reduce the panic caused by the false belief that "everyone's doing it," to emphasize the unfavorable consequences of premarital promiscuity, and to stress the freedoms and benefits associated with a lifestyle of self-control.

Schools must forsake their current hypocrisy about parental involvement in sex education. On the one hand, schools are always using parental irresponsibility as the primary justification for teaching sex education in school, while on the other hand, doing everything they can to discourage parental input, knowledge, and participation in the formulation and teaching of sex education courses.

Schools simply must take effective measures to foster greater parental involvement in sex education. Traditional contraceptive-oriented sex education programs are designed to exclude parents and to convince students that parents are irrelevant. These courses stress that the decision to have sexual intercourse must be the student's own decision, according to his or her own value system, and they emphasize that students can get birth control, venereal disease treatment, and abortions without parental knowledge or consent. So much for fostering greater parental involvement.

In contrast to the traditional contraceptive-oriented sex education courses, the new chastity-based curriculums are designed to encourage maximum parental participation. The *Sex Respect*[7] curriculum, for instance, provides a curriculum guide for the teacher, a textbook for the student, and a parents' guide. The parents' guide provides an overview of the course and provides specific guidelines to help the parents supplement the classroom teaching by providing direction and confidence in helping teens understand their human sexuality. The parents' guide also helps parents understand the causes and dynamics of peer pressure, the effects of social pressure, media, music, and dating, and it helps the parents formulate sensible steps to aid their children in resisting bad peer pressure, dangerous sexual situations and behaviors, and decisions that limit life options.

Schools can also reduce premarital teen promiscuity and pregnancy by doing a better job of motivating and educating students. Both national and international studies have uncovered the influence of despair, academic failure, and economic, academic, and emotional deprivation in exacerbating the teen pregnancy problem.

The media are a thornier problem. Nevertheless, the media do respond to public pressure and to social trends, and there is no reason to believe that the American media must get progressively filthier throughout eternity. The alternative to filthy television is cleaner television. In the short term, the alternative to filthy media is a flick of the wrist. Scientific studies show that turning off the television or the radio rarely proves fatal.

If parents and churches and schools and teens will do their part, America will not need to look to the government for some massive compulsory sex education or compulsory birth control program, nor will we have provided the government and Planned Parenthood the excuse for such programs. The price of liberty is eternal vigilance.

---

7. Authored by Colleen Kelly Mast and partially funded by the federal government, *Sex Respect: The Option of True Sexual Freedom* (Bradley, IL: Respect, Inc., 1986) is in use in hundreds of public schools across the United States. The *Sex Respect* curriculum is particularly effective in reducing premarital pregnancy and promiscuity partly because it emphatically involves parents in the program.

Summary

America is a nation divided between two visions of the future, a vision of life and a vision of death. The approach we take on sex education, contraception, and teen pregnancy will determine whether America lives or dies — culturally, spiritually, and demographically.

Planned Parenthood is winning the battle for our children's minds and souls, and it will continue to win until we render it irrelevant, and that means that we must begin to train our children in chastity and a lifestyle of self-control.

We must replace our schools' amoral, situational ethics-based, contraceptive-oriented sex education programs with chastity-based curricula such as *Sex Respect*. And we must begin *now* to implement *Sex Respect* in schools that have no sex education curriculum.

We can continue to allow Planned Parenthood to define the issue and propose its self-serving, secular, and anti-religious "solutions," solutions guaranteed to cleanse America of the last vestiges of Christian influence and traditional Western morality, or we can start now to fulfill our God-ordained responsibilities as parents, churches, and schools. We can provide our children the *vision* and the *values* needed to steer them safely through adolescence and to happy marriages and happy families.

EIGHT

TEEN PREGNANCY: FINDING SOLUTIONS

Teen promiscuity, especially among minors, is aberrational. The magnitude of the teen pregnancy problem has been greatly inflated by Planned Parenthood's hype.

More importantly, premarital teen pregnancy is solvable. We have shown that teen pregnancy is primarily the result of peer pressure and social pressure. It is simply a myth to say that unmarried teens have sex because they are in love, or that they have sex because they have uncontrollable biological urges. We can reduce teen fornication because we can change the atmosphere that influences teens to devalue virginity and to feel pressured to "do it."

Before we can really attack teen pregnancy, we need to acknowledge a few foundational realities:

1. Teen fornication can never be totally eradicated, nor can we ever eliminate *all* pregnancies to unmarried teens. We can vigorously discourage rape and murder through strong laws, good law enforcement, and widespread social condemnation, but we cannot totally eliminate rape and murder; neither can we totally eliminate teen fornication. There will always be a small number of teens who will have sex before marriage and who will get pregnant. This has been true in all societies at all times, whether in Egypt five thousand years ago, Jerusalem at 100 B.C., or America today. Neither the chastity approach nor the birth control approach to teen pregnancy can ever totally eradicate the problem. The best we can hope for is to hold down the problem to the residual level.

2. When we speak of teens, we are speaking of a group of people who get older by the minute. Teens grow up and are no

longer teen-agers, and new teen-agers take their places. Thus, to discuss teen-agers in 1987 and teen-agers in 1994 is to discuss two *entirely different* sets of people. This is a very obvious fact that is often overlooked, but its implications are enormous, in fact, *enormously encouraging*. Why? Because oftentimes people insist that the chastity and peer pressure reduction approach is unrealistic because some teens are already promiscuous, and these teens cannot be expected to simply postpone further sexual intercourse until marriage. The chastity approach is said to abandon these teens. But this attitude ignores two realities: (1) The birth control approach has been used for over twenty years, with no success. It abandons teens who prefer chastity but need lifestyle reinforcement, peer encouragement, and mentor exhortation, and (2) The chastity approach is applicable to the vast majority of teens because the vast majority of teens are still virgins, and within six years, this approach could be fully functioning throughout an entirely new set of teens. *Thus, even if 100% of all teens were sexually active today, that would not imply that we should therefore abandon all future teen-agers to the same fate.* Because teens are not a static group, rates of teen intercourse are not static. Nineteen-year-old teens, many of whom have had sex, are yearly replaced by new thirteen-year-old teens, very few of whom have had sex.

It should be noted that any approach to teen pregnancy must start with a definition of the problem. Planned Parenthood defines teen pregnancy as problematic, without regard to marital status. Planned Parenthood's concern with teen pregnancy ranges from a heavy condemnation of teen births, to alarm at teen pregnancy, to almost no concern for teen promiscuity.

This approach is all wrong. First, teen pregnancy is not the problem; to define it as such is to disparage marriage. If married teen-agers want to have sex and have babies, that's perfectly moral and wonderful, and it is perverted for Planned Parenthood and the U.S. government to define such healthy family creation as problematic.

Teen births are not the problem.[1] To define the problem as

---

1. The problem is not teen abortions, either. Teen abortions are inexcusable, but even if we could eliminate all teen abortions, we would still be left with teen fornication and teen cohabitation and teen illegitimate childbirth, and these behaviors should also be discouraged as unhealthy to teens and to society as a whole.

births, whether to married or unmarried teens, is an implicitly pro-abortion viewpoint. *To attack teen births rather than teen pregnancy is to attack innocent babies rather than immoral behaviors.*

The problem is teen fornication. To focus on anything else is to focus on results and consequences rather than on behaviors. That focus will inevitably lead us to seek technical, nonmoral solutions. But sexual behavior is a moral issue. Fornication is a sin, and because it is a sin, it produces undesirable consequences. But it is foolish and unrealistic to define the curses as problematic rather than the accursed behavior that spawned the undesirable results.

When we accurately define the problem, the solutions become clear. The birth control approach is a failed attempt to mitigate the fallout from sexual sin by technical or medical means. The birth control approach says nothing about sexual behavior, only about technical behavior: "You should use this device when you have sex with your partner."

The birth control approach is too narrow, too disjointed, because it ignores the spiritual and emotional aspects of teen intercourse. But teen fornication has important spiritual and emotional consequences that cannot be ignored, because teens are neither machines nor mere animals. Teens are fully human; they have a spirit and a soul as well as a body. Birth control treats only the body. The birth control approach is suitable for dogs and cats but is an inhuman approach to the sexual behavior of God's greatest creation, a creation that has spiritual and emotional dimensions which far transcend the body, but which are also inextricably linked with the body. To ignore the spiritual and emotional dimensions of our behavior is to demand that we function as only part-human—the animal part.

We have been told that the sex education/contraceptive education/sex clinic approach to teen pregnancy is comprehensive and realistic. But it's not. How can we call this approach comprehensive when it completely ignores religion, morality, law, tradition, history, spirituality, emotion, and venereal disease?

Clearly, the birth control approach to teen pregnancy is the wrong solution to the wrong problem.

Chastity is the only approach to teen fornication (or teen pregnancies or teen births or teen abortions) that is truly comprehensive. The lifestyle of chastity is a healthy one that promotes a realistic, holistic, whole-person approach to sex, rather than treating sexual behavior as a totally isolated and autonomous sphere of action.

The lifestyle of chastity is one of self-control, not self-gratification. It reinforces abstinence from sexual behavior by promoting abstinence from all harmful behaviors: The chaste individual practices self-control in eating, in drinking alcohol, in abstaining from illegal drugs, and he or she practices discretion in deciding what movies to watch, what magazines to read, and what clothes to wear. The chaste individual is willing to sacrifice present pleasure for future gain, in direct contrast to the birth-control teen-ager who is willing to risk ruining his or her future for the sake of immediate sexual gratification.

Both chastity-based sex education and contraceptive-based sex education require training rather than the mere transmission of knowledge in order for them to affect teens. But contraceptive behavior cannot be safely or effectively taught: You can teach the proper use of contraceptives, but to get even a moderate level of teens to translate this knowledge into actual practice requires consistent reinforcement and exhortation and persuasion. Unfortunately, while consistency in contraceptive behavior is being taught to sexually active teens, many of them are getting pregnant.

Fortunately, chastity-based sex education's training is not so dangerous. Chastity education, too, requires much more than merely teaching some facts in a classroom. Like contraceptive training, chastity training requires reinforcement, encouragement, and exhortation, but unlike contraceptive training, the training period is not automatically fraught with urgent dangers.

We as a society must abandon the absurd notion that premarital teen promiscuity or pregnancy can be controlled by teaching a one-hour course five days a week. *Teen pregnancy is not a true-false subject.* It is the result of wrong behavior, not wrong answers on a pop quiz. It is not the inevitable result of sexual ignorance, or of not having had a formal sex education course. Premarital teen pregnancy is the result of bad moral choices.

If all premarital teen pregnancy were truly the result of a failure to receive contraceptive sex education, then the teen illegitimate pregnancy problem would have raged until the late 1960s and then died out as students began receiving formal sex education and contraceptive education.[2] But even though the overwhelming majority of students today have received formal sex education, and even though the overwhelming majority of sexually active teens already use birth control (whereas fifty or one hundred years ago very few received formal sex/contraceptive education or used birth control), the teen pregnancy crisis is a post-1960 problem. If sex education, free government-paid birth control for all unemancipated minors, contraceptive education, and "values clarification" were the answers to premarital teen pregnancy, then by 1988, the teen pregnancy problem should have been reduced tremendously from historical levels.

The great increase in teen promiscuity and premarital pregnancy that occurred during the 1960s and early 1970s was not the result of students' not having had sex education or access to contraception. The increases were the result of a profound reversal of the societal and peer pressure not to engage in premarital intercourse:[3] Instead of pressure to confine sexual intercourse to acts between two married persons, there developed a pressure to engage in sexual intercourse premaritally, and to a lesser degree, extramaritally. "If it feels good, do it!" became the slogan of a generation that had rejected the traditional sexual restraints of Western culture.

The social and cultural barriers to premarital and extramarital sexual intercourse had always been much stronger in America than the explicitly religious barriers. The threat of a ruined rep-

---

2. According to *American Teens Speak*, 60% of all American teenagers report having received formal sex education in school.

3. For instance, *Family Planning Perspectives* published this analysis of teen pregnancy rates for 1971-1979: "Furthermore, young women appear to be having less success in avoiding accidental pregnancies than in preventing unplanned births. Even though more teenagers are using contraceptives, and more of them are using birth control methods consistently, pregnancy rates have continued to climb. . . . This discouraging situation is highlighted by the fact that although nonuse of contraceptive methods has declined in recent years, the fall has not been sufficient to overcome the forces that are working to elevate pregnancy rates. . . ." Melvin Zelnick and John F. Kantner, "Sexual Activity, Contraceptive Use and Pregnancy Among Metropolitan-Area Teenagers: 1971-1979," *Family Planning Perspectives* 12:5 (September/October, 1980).

utation was always a greater incentive to sexual morality than the fires of Hell ever were, and Heaven never had the tangible certainty of satisfaction that intercourse seemed to promise.

Traditional and cultural mores and taboos came under sharp attack during the 1960s as the under-thirty generation rejected racism and patriotism, the former out of love for fellow man, and the latter out of love of self. But the whole culture of rock music and drugs and the heady excitement of ushering in a whole new age founded on peace, love, and tolerance, all of which had been invented by them (so they thought), led to a rejection of traditional sexual mores as well.

Nevertheless, a widespread personal rejection probably would not have happened without an almost universal belief that the invention of the birth control pill had rendered all sex safe from unintended pregnancy — in fact, safe in general.[4] Thus, a personal plunge into sexual hedonism and adventurism seemed to hold little risk and the promise of much reward.

Two other premises that underlay the rejection of traditional sexual mores were the belief that any behavior was acceptable as long as it did not directly harm another person unwillingly, and the belief that traditional sexual mores were designed to discriminate against women and "keep them in their proper place."

Realistic people no longer accept these premises. First, the Pill has a significant failure rate, and it provides zero protection against AIDS or any other venereal disease. Second, private acts have public consequences, as the AIDS crisis and abortion and pornography have taught us. And third, the Sexual Revolution liberated men, not women. Men (to use the term loosely) walked out on their wives and children, abandoning them to a life of poverty and despair. Meanwhile, the irresponsible male's disposable income soared, and he enjoyed the liberty of responsibility-free sex with a huge selection of women. Women got liberated from alimony and child support.

Things change. Today, no one seriously tries to pass off marijuana as a serious means to expand artistic ability or creativity.

---

4. The threat of venereal disease was not considered significant since venereal disease had always been confined mostly to syphilis and gonorrhea, both of which had been rendered harmless by the discovery of penicillin. Incurable venereal diseases such as herpes and AIDS were more or less unknown.

No one seriously advocates LSD as a way to expand your consciousness and get your life together. The Vietnamese boat people and the invasion of Afghanistan dissolved the self-delusion that communism was a benign people's movement. Hippies became yuppies. The ERA was defeated, largely by middle-class housewives.

It is clear that the teen promiscuity and premarital pregnancy problem developed as a direct result of a loosening of social pressure and peer pressure. It is equally clear that the sex education/contraceptive education approach is a narrow technical approach that has proved ineffective at either eliminating consequences or changing behavior for the good.

The contraceptive approach to teen pregnancy has no hope of succeeding as long as contraceptive use remains voluntary rather than mandatory, and as long as persuasion is employed rather than coercion. *Sexually irresponsible teens are also sexually irresponsible contraceptors.* We cannot expect *all* teens to *always* use contraception any more than we can expect *all* teens to *always* clean their rooms, make their beds, brush their teeth, or drive within speed limits. Teens are notoriously unreliable contraceptors. Some teens will never voluntarily use contraception, and many others will never use it consistently, every time. This is just human nature.

The advocates of contraception for teens are well aware that coercion is necessary if they are to demonstrate progress. One integral rationale for placing contraceptive-dispensing sex clinics in the schools is that dispensing contraceptives on site affords the clinic personnel the ability to monitor the contraceptive behavior of the clients. But there is a fine line between persuasion and coercion.

Indeed, proponents of birth control have for decades openly advocated coercive and totalitarian approaches to fertility control. These approaches have included appeals for licensing of parents, for forced sterilization (minority groups, mentally or physically disadvantaged people, ethnic groups, parents with more than two children, etc.), and for criminal sanctions for "overpopulaters." For instance, Edgar R. Chasteen, a founding member of Zero Population Growth, Inc., and a board member of Planned Parenthood Association of Greater Kansas City, wrote a book entitled *The Case for Compulsory Birth Control* in which he advocated governmental repeal of parents' rights to bear children through the passage of the following law:

Public Law Number ---,
Reversible Fertility Immunization

As of January 1, 1975 it shall be unlawful for any American family to give birth to more than two children. Any family already having two or more natural children on that date shall not be allowed to give birth to another. Toward this end, it is hereby lawfully determined that *all* Americans above the age of 10 years will, at least one year prior to the aforementioned date present himself/herself for reversible immunization against fertility at a local county health department or physician's office. An official "Certificate of Immunization" shall be issued to and in the name of each citizen so treated. Said certification shall be signed by the authorized medical practitioner who administers the immunization and shall be entered into the official records of the county in which immunization occurred. After marriage, any citizen may present himself/herself at a local county health department or physician's office and obtain a fertility restorer. At the birth of the second child, immunity against fertility shall be readministered to both parents. If the first birth shall be multiple, no other births shall be permitted to that mother, and both parents shall thereupon be re-immunized.[5]

Welcome to Planned Parenthood's Amerika, comrade!

Chasteen recognized that contraception and human nature were at cross purposes and that to succeed on a macro scale, contraception would have to be coercive, aimed at changing behavior and controlling behavior:

Some future historian will look back on the twentieth century and write that in the year 19--, laws were passed in America which struck down forever that anachronistic practice to which we had too long adhered—the right to have as many children as we wanted. That "want" after all is socially created and may be socially redefined. No one is born wanting a certain number of children any more than one wants at birth to speak English

---

5. Edgar R. Chasteen, *The Case For Compulsory Birth Control* (Englewood Cliffs, NJ: Prentice-Hall, 1971).

or to eat with a fork. The desire to give birth to one, four, seven or fifteen children is thus exposed for what it is — an accident — conditioned by the time and place of our own birth. That future historian will consider us uncivilized for having permitted unregulated births as we do the Romans and Chinese for their "irresponsible" behavior.[6]

According to Chasteen, Zero Population Growth, Inc., passed the following resolutions at its September 1969 board meeting:

1. It is resolved that parenthood is not an inherent right of individuals but a privilege extended by the society in which they live. Accordingly, society has both the right and the duty to limit population when either its physical existence or its quality of life is threatened.

2. We further resolve that every American family is entitled to give birth to children, but no family has the right to have more than two children.

3. We further resolve that the Congress of the United States must (a) enact legislation guaranteeing the right of parenthood to all Americans but restricting the number of natural (not adoptive) children to two, and (b) adopt and finance a "crash" program to develop a birth control technology sufficient to accomplish this objective without using criminal sanctions.[7]

It is interesting to note that Chasteen wrote *The Case for Compulsory Birth Control* as well-to-do, scholarly father of *three* children:

My concern is not for myself, for I have been singularly fortunate in acquiring a loving wife, three fine, healthy children and the only job I ever wanted — that of a teacher. My personal ambition has been satisfied, but my public anxiety increases with each day's headlines.[8]

Chasteen is highly educated, with a secure job and a comfortable income. He considers himself "fortunate" to have *three* children, and he expresses no apology or anxiety or remorse for having three children

---

6. Ibid., p. 84.
7. Ibid., p. 94.
8. Ibid., p. viii.

while advocating the jailing of parents who intentionally birth more than two.[9] Although Chasteen claims a total lack of self-interest, the book is replete with paranoic ranting that the welfare of the rich and powerful is being threatened by overpopulation:

> . . . If that is true, and there is little to suggest that it is not, then all the world is about to be engulfed by horrors beyond description. These doomed nations [India and others] will not slip quietly into history. As their condition and its ultimate conclusion becomes clearer to them, they will lash out blindly and irrationally in a last desperate attempt to save themselves. Failing at this, their final act will be to ensure that other nations, particularly the rich and powerful ones, die with them.[10]

Interestingly, Chasteen prescribes compulsory U.S. population control programs to be forced upon all recipients of U.S. foreign aid. Unfortunately, his suggestion has become reality.

Chasteen is exceptional among organized family planning advocates not in his extremist views, but in his willingness to publicly advocate them. The entire organized birth control movement has been dominated by coercive utopians from the beginning.

Coercion is not the only offensive looming danger in the contraceptive approach to teen pregnancy. It is interesting to note that the example of Sweden is regularly hailed as exemplary. Sweden, in fact, does have teen pregnancy and abortion rates that are about half those of the United States. But that is true of just about every other major country, including Canada, England, France, and the Netherlands. In fact, the Netherlands has teen pregnancy and abortion rates that are less than one-fifth as great as in the United States (and less than half as great as the rates in Sweden). Not only does the Netherlands have by far the lowest teen pregnancy and abortion rates, but also, of those teens who do get pregnant, it has the highest percentage of legitimate births, the lowest percentage of abortions, and the lowest percentage of illegitimate births.

So why do they always point to Sweden as the success story and role model for the United States?

The answer is to be found in how Planned Parenthood and other organized family planning groups define "success." Gener-

---

9. Ibid., p. 209.
10. Ibid., prologue.

ally, they regard any approach to teen pregnancy as successful if it involves a greater role for family planning clinics. Remember Faye Wattleton's remark that 9.5 million American teens "remain unserved" because they are not customers of government-funded family planning clinics?

It does not matter that Sweden has a higher abortion rate than the entire teen pregnancy rate in the Netherlands. It does not matter that Sweden has the highest rate of teen sexual intercourse of any country studied.[11] What matters is that Sweden's approach to sex education, if mimicked by the United States, would result in a huge expansion of government funding for Planned Parenthood:

> By and large, of all the countries studied, Sweden has been the most active in developing programs and policies to reduce teen pregnancy. These efforts include universal education in sexuality and contraception; development of special clinics — closely associated with the schools — where young people receive contraceptive services and counseling; free, widely available and confidential contraceptive and abortion services; widespread advertising of contraceptives in all media; frank treatment of sex; and availability of condoms from a variety of sources.[12]

But the choice of Sweden is not motivated solely by organizational survival and economic self-interest; the choice is also ideological, because Sweden is an example of a country that has adopted a completely secular, amoral approach to teen pregnancy. Teens in Sweden have been liberated to full sexual enjoyment.

Indeed, the advocates of the contraceptive approach to teen pregnancy do not view teen premarital promiscuity as undesirable.[13] This

---

11. Sweden was the first country in the world to mandate compulsory sex education in schools. This sex education is required through all grade levels. Sweden has the highest rate of teen sexual activity, significantly higher even than that of the United States. On the other hand, the Netherlands has no formal sex education other than the teaching of the biological facts of reproduction in science classes. The Netherlands has a far lower rate of first-time teen sexual intercourse than Sweden.

12. Elise F. Jones, et al., p. 61.

13. They view teen parenthood, in or out of wedlock, planned or unplanned, as undesirable. They view teen abortion as generally desirable, certainly desirable compared to the alternative of parenthood, especially if the conception was due to contraceptive failure.

conclusion is self-evident from their whole approach to defining and combatting teen pregnancy, but it is also a conclusion documented by research. In her book *Abortion and the Politics of Motherhood*, Kristin Luker presents research into the worldviews of pro-life and pro-choice activists. She says:

> Connected to this value [family planning] is an acceptance of teen-aged sex. Pro-choice people are concerned about teen-aged *parenthood* because young people and the unwed are in no position to become good parents, but they have no basic objection to sexual activity among young people *if they are "responsible,"* that is, if they do not take the risk of becoming parents. Because pro-choice people view the goal of sex as being the creation of intimacy, caring, and trust, they also believe that people need to practice those skills before making a long-term commitment to someone. They may practice them with a number of people or with the person they intend to marry. In either case, premarital sex is not only likely to occur, but desirable.[14]

America stands at a crossroads. It can become Swedenized, or it can return to traditional standards of morality, chastity, and proper behavior. It seems clear that the contraceptive approach to teen pregnancy has little hope of succeeding unless we are ready to regard increased promiscuity and coercive birth control practices as "successes." Even if the contraceptive approach were to be embraced, the social costs alone would almost surely ruin the nation (not to mention the teen-agers themselves): Every European nation studied as a model of contraceptive success has a national birthrate below the replacement level. All are dying nations. Sweden, the darling of the coercive utopians, has a birthrate more than forty percent below the replacement level. Sweden is dying fast.

The totalitarian approach to teen pregnancy, such as employed in Sweden, is neither appropriate nor desirable nor necessary for the United States. The United States has the freedom to pursue a much more comprehensive approach to teen pregnancy, promiscuity, and premarital sex, an approach that is consistent with life and health and preparing for marriage and families and careers.[15]

---

14. Luker, pp. 182-183.

15. For a comprehensive but concise discussion of this topic, see Allan Carlson, "Pregnant Teenagers and Moral Civil Wars," *Human Life Review* 11:4 (New York: The Human Life Foundation, Inc., Fall 1985).

Premarital teen pregnancy is solvable, because teen promiscuity is primarily a peer pressure/social pressure problem. We can reduce premarital teen pregnancy because we can reduce peer pressure, reinforce teens' majority choices to live chaste lifestyles, and mitigate or reduce social pressure.

We need to forsake the misguided belief in the efficacy of traditional sex education. The sterile transmission of information about sex, whether that information is biological or contraceptive-oriented or chastity-oriented, cannot hope to have a significant positive influence on teen sexual behavior. What we need is a more comprehensive view of sex education, a view that acknowledges that true sex education involves training and exampling and exhorting and encouraging as a process, rather than the mere transmission of information.

It would be severely misguided to believe that merely teaching teen-agers about chastity, about the failures and dangers of birth control, and about the wonderful purpose of sex, would be sufficient to immunize teens against premarital intercourse. What is needed is a view of sex education that is holistic and which is geared toward training and reinforcement rather than accumulation of knowledge.

This more expansive and realistic view of sex education teaches chastity and healthy sexual purity as one integral aspect of a lifestyle of chastity whereby teens learn and practice self-control in all areas of their lives: They learn to say no to drugs, to avoid overdrinking, to sacrifice short-term pleasure for the sake of long-term goals, to control their sexual behavior, to respect their own bodies and to respect women's bodies, and to respect the awesome power of procreation.

We need to give teen-agers both positive and negative reasons to avoid premarital and extramarital sex. The all-too-often traditional view of chastity that views proper sex education as being summed up by, "Don't do it until you're married," is a flawed and insufficient view of sex education. *Chastity training is not synonymous with listing sixty-eight rules restricting promiscuity.*

We must communicate both positive and negative reasons why sex should be confined to marriage. We must transmit a coherent, unified vision of sex that extols the positive benefits of chastity, emphasizes the certain curses and dangers of promiscuity, and provides explicit guidelines for behavior. We need to convey to teens that self-control is a positive protective and life-enriching behavior, not just a way to avoid fun.

We must communicate to teens that sex is purposeful rather than purely recreational. If sex were intended solely for pleasure, then there would be no necessity for confining sex to marriage. But sex is not solely intended for pleasure, nor is it primarily intended for pleasure.

Sexual intercourse is the mechanism of procreation, and we ignore this biological fact at our own peril. The fundamental purpose of sex is procreation, not recreation.[16] Because children deserve families, sexual intercourse belongs within marriage.

But there is an aspect of sexual intercourse that transcends the procreative purpose. This aspect involves intimacy and physical, spiritual, and emotional sharing and unity, a sort of bonding. But Scripture informs us that this bonding was also intended solely within the marriage (Genesis, chapters 2 and 3). A close sexual relationship can provoke a deep bonding which, when broken off, is as painful as a divorce.

We must also communicate to teens that procreation is not evil. Planned Parenthood's approach to intercourse treats pregnancy and childbirth as life's worst curses. We must emphasize the truth that procreation is a marvelous, miraculous act, as is childbirth. The conception and birth of a baby is a tremendous miracle that man cannot duplicate, only manipulate. The "facts of life" are miraculous facts.

If we cannot tell teens that sex is more than just recreation, we cannot hope to reduce teen promiscuity. Planned Parenthood's greatest triumph has been to reduce the beauty and power and sacredness of sexual intercourse to a mere recreational act.

Parents, not schools, are the keys to proper sex education. Parents have tremendous powers of influence and persuasion over

16. This is not to say that all sexual acts must be deliberately procreative, but it is to acknowledge that our sexual organs were given to us for procreation. Likewise, our digestive systems were given to us for eating, and although eating is pleasurable, no one argues that the elemental purpose of eating is pleasure. If we eat only junk food, we die; we cannot deny the nutritive purpose of eating.

their children, and parents can help foster an atmosphere that encourages and reinforces chaste behavior in all areas of life. In sex education, schools should be used as tools to reinforce parental training rather than as substitutes for parental responsibility.

Parents should help teens value their virginity and should inculcate a desire to avoid harmful behaviors. Do you want your child to have premarital sex? Fine, do nothing. Let them listen to any filthy music, watch any perverted movie, hang around with promiscuous friends, use drugs, and persist in sub-optimal performance in school. Let them raise themselves. And then you can raise your grandchildren for them.

Parents can influence peer pressure by helping their teens to choose good friends and develop good patterns of self-control. Churches and parents can communicate a consistent and comprehensive vision of sexual behavior and its consequences. Schools can reinforce abstinence and healthy lifestyles. Peer pressure can be reduced.

But what about societal pressures? What about the pervasive negative influence of television, movies, magazines, music? Well, the solution offered by Planned Parenthood is to admit defeat and then to call for more negative societal pressure. Planned Parenthood has been waging a sometimes successful campaign to sterilize filthy American airwaves by promoting contraceptive advertising and the portrayal of contracepted sex.

Planned Parenthood wants to Swedenize America, to turn us into a sex-and-contraception-saturated nation. Yes, American television is filthy and perverted, and its unrealistic portrayal of consequence-free sex does aggravate premarital promiscuity. But the alternative to filth and failure and irresponsibility is not more filth and failure and irresponsibility, but less. What do they want *Hustler* magazine to do? Show naked women with little arrows pointing to the approximate location of their IUDs? Wouldn't that be a step forward? Why don't we get X-rated movie stars to slap on a condom first? Wouldn't that make a dent in premarital pregnancy?

As a society, we must return to a high regard for children, not as life enrichment units, not as successful students, not as potential college graduates, not as potential lawyers and bankers, not as future citizens and taxpayers, but as persons made in the image of God, creatures with eternal souls and intrinsic value and worth. When we see children as truly valuable gifts from God, when we acknowledge our responsibility to raise them with care and love and moral guidance, we will also return to shielding and protecting them from dangerous influences and situations until they are emotionally and morally equipped to handle them and to make the right choices. Childhood should once again become a period of joy, joy that springs from innocence, rather than a period of persistent brutalization by a wicked, perverse adult world.

It is not enough to simply halt the teaching of immoral and dangerous Planned Parenthood-style sex education programs in our schools. We must go further. We must place chastity programs such as *Sex Respect* in our schools, and parents and churches must begin to directly train children in proper sexual knowledge, beliefs, attitudes, and behavior. It is not enough to merely thwart the teaching of sexual immorality; we must fill the void with correct instruction.

Planned Parenthood knows that the battle over sex education is a battle for whose moral code will shape the minds of all future Americans. Planned Parenthood is the main proponent of K-12 compulsory comprehensive contraceptive-oriented sex education. The fundamental question is whether we will abandon our children, and our nation's future, to the failed educational perversions of the coercive utopians, or whether we will return to moral sanity and inculcate healthy, moral, life-affirming values in our children.

Teen pregnancy is solvable. The choice is ours.

NINE

ABORTING PLANNED PARENTHOOD: STRATEGIES

Though it is exceedingly large and powerful, Planned Parenthood is also quite vulnerable. Its programs are disasters: Its birth control doesn't work; its abortions aren't safe and healthful; its endorsement of promiscuity leads to the spread of incurable and fatal venereal diseases; its racist programs rape taxpayers.

No matter what aspect of its operations, history or goals you analyze, Planned Parenthood is vulnerable. Even its financial success could prove disastrous: Planned Parenthood Federation of America had built up such large cash reserves by 1986, it feared that potential donors would not respond to its fear-mongering appeals that "reproductive freedom is in greater danger today than ever before."[1]

We can slay the dragon. We can shut off the torrent of tax-payer subsidies. We can educate school boards about the dangers of its sex education and birth control programs. We can help wounded women recover legal damages against its clinics and doctors.

But even if we were to successfully liberate America (and the American taxpayer) from the oppressive scourge of Planned Parenthood, would we have done enough? Is fervent opposition to this destructive and deadly organization all that is required of us?

The answer, of course, is no.

Opposing Planned Parenthood will certainly help prevent America from getting worse; it will not, however, do enough to

---

1. Refer to the minutes of the October 17, 1986 PPFA Board of Directors meeting in which this fear was exhaustively discussed and analyzed.

make America better. Our opposition to Planned Parenthood is absolutely *necessary*; it is not, however, *sufficient*.

Our opposition must be balanced by active efforts to promote positive alternatives. So, for instance, rather than merely opposing Planned Parenthood-style sex education programs, we should simultaneously work to implement moral, life-affirming sex education programs in school and churches.

In schools, in churches, in community groups, in crisis pregnancy centers, we must begin to work to make Planned Parenthood irrelevant. We must use these institutions to transmit to our youth and our society a clear vision of sexual health and success. We must no longer remain silent about sexuality.

By maintaining a balance between educational efforts and purely oppositional tactics, we will ensure that we avoid the primary cause of burnout: frustration. Our opposition to Planned Parenthood will undoubtedly continue to be difficult and fraught with temporary setbacks. We will be able to avoid burnout and disillusionment and fatigue if we are constantly buoyed by the knowledge that we are making a difference in teens' lives — in a real life, face to face manner — through our moral sex education efforts in schools and churches.

We would be making a terrible mistake to adopt any strategy of opposition that is not balanced by reaching teens in some forum with facts and instruction and encouragement and exhortation and exampling in how to live successful, healthy and moral lives in all areas, including their sex lives. Teen-agers will not learn the right way and the best way and the healthy way to live by mere osmosis or by being kept ignorant. It is up to us to make the real difference in their lives.

We must remember that Planned Parenthood has always had a three-pronged strategy involving clinics, schools, and churches. There are already over two hundred Planned Parenthood affiliates and seven hundred Planned Parenthood clinics nationwide, and its sex education programs are pervasive among our schools, both public and private. It is clear, then, that Planned Parenthood's next real thrust will be to establish itself as a credible part of church ministries.

The real danger is that we might fail to initiate good, moral, life-affirming sex education programs in our churches, choosing instead to devote *all* of our energies and resources to just fighting in arenas where we have, largely, already lost—in the schools and at the clinics. If we allow Planned Parenthood's sex education programs to infiltrate our churches as they have our schools, we will find ourselves in almost hopeless straits. If we are shut out of government programs, schools, and churches, what other organized, credible forums would we have to espouse sane views of sexuality? None.

That is why the first and foremost our opposition to Planned Parenthood must concentrate on churches, not clinics, not schools. We must establish solid sex education programs in churches, and oppose any vestigial sympathies to the Planned Parenthood "sex-is-right-if-it's-right-for-*you*" philosophy.[2]

Tactics of Opposition

Okay, okay. You're already teaching moral sex education at home, at church, and at the Boy Scouts hall, and what you really want to do now is directly oppose Planned Parenthood. So what do you do?

Obviously, the appropriate tactics vary depending on the level targeted and the resources and talents of the activists. Nevertheless, no single tactic and no single level is more important than another. If we are to be successful, we must hit Planned Parenthood at every level with every type of tactic. We have the manpower and the ability to cripple Planned Parenthood, and now we also have the tools and the strategy to get the job done.

National

On the national level, we must demand that Congress reform the Title XX program to sever Planned Parenthood's incestuous relationship with federal and state population program administrative agencies and to stop Planned Parenthood's rape of the taxpayer. The present administration of Title XX funds is a fraud and a scam, and we must insist that Congress fix the problem by effective legislation.

---

2. Life Advocates in Houston, Texas publishes an excellent sex education curriculum for churches. Write to Life Advocates, One West Loop South, Suite 811, Houston, Texas 77027. Videotape and cassette tapes are also available.

Congress must:

1. Reinstate accountability for the spending of Title XX funds. States must be required to submit detailed spending plans and then to prove that they spent the funds in accordance with those plans.

2. Outlaw contracts with providers who:
   a. Charge higher rates for government-funded patients than for cash patients. The taxpayer should not have to pay $500.00 for a $5.00 hammer, nor $57.18 for a "free" pregnancy test.
   b. Charge higher average billings (for any particular purpose of visit) for government-funded clients than for cash clients. Government-paid clients must not be used as tools for pumping up revenues and profits by billing unnecessary service or by charging for services that are provided free to cash clients.

   These rules must apply both to contracts administered at the federal level and to contracts administered at the state level. In fact, Title XX funds should be withheld from any state that does not implement these regulations and an effective enforcement procedure at the state level. (Yes, you can do that: States who refused to raise their drinking age to twenty-one were denied federal highway funds.)

3. Require written parental consent for unmarried minors to obtain prescription contraceptive chemicals or devices.

4. Restore income eligibility determination and verification requirements. Income must be defined as income from all sources, and it should include parents' income for any unemancipated minor. Income eligibility must be verified and documented in a manner similar to Medicaid, and must be done at the government level, not at the clinic level.

5. Prohibit the use of Title XX funds for providing prescription contraceptives to unmarried persons. Dispensing prescription contraceptives to unmarried persons is contrary to public health and results in a government subsidy of, and incentive to, dangerous and undesirable behavior. This would not outlaw the dispensing of contraceptives to unmarried persons, but it would get government out of the business of encouraging and subsidizing immoral and life-threatening behaviors. It would have the dual effect of discouraging promiscuity and encouraging condom usage

(since condoms are extremely cheap and easy to obtain), which is safer than nonbarrier methods of contraception (although still not safe).

These measures represent interim goals only. Our ultimate goal would be to prohibit the use of federal funds for family planning services. The Title V and XX programs were never intended to be used as vehicles to shovel money to Planned Parenthood so that it could exacerbate the AIDS epidemic and the teen pregnancy problem while claiming to be serving the indigent and needy.

We must also demand that Congress end the Title X debacle. Congress must:

1. Restore accountability to the federal government for how states and other grantees or contract recipients expend family planning funds.

2. Outlaw the dispensing of Title X funds to any organization or program that presents fornication as responsible behavior, that teaches that sex outside of marriage can be totally safe or as safe as chastity, or that does not teach chastity as the only safe and preferred lifestyle for unmarried people. Government must be removed from endorsing or sponsoring programs that encourage dangerous and unsafe behavior.

3. Ensure that Title X grants require at least 50% matching state funds. Presently they require only 10%.

4. Remove the requirement that Title X funds may go only to organizations that counsel or refer for abortions. Title X funds must be explicitly allowed to go exclusively to organizations that provide only nonabortion-related maternal diagnosis and help services such as adoption.

Congress must also prohibit the dispensing of Title V, X, XIX, or XX funds to any organization that offers discounts, incentives, gifts, prizes, or contests for Medicaid or government-funded clients. In addition, Congress must prohibit federal funding of any organization or program that targets any religious, ethnic, racial, national, or income-level group for family planning or abortion. The federal government must stop bankrolling racism, xenophobia, and genocide under the guise of family planning.

All of these strategies are good, but we also need to re-evaluate our relationship to certain pervasive political beliefs.

First, we need to remember that the blessings of God are given in return for obedience to God's laws, not for having the "proper" form of government. God's blessings upon a nation are dispensed in return for obedience and faithfulness, not for setting up a system of checks and balances or a separation of powers. What matters to God is obedience to just laws, not what governmental system develops and enforces those laws.

It really does not matter what the intent was of the Founding Fathers. What if they intended homosexual rape to be legal? Would that make it right? If we believe in "original intent," must we not also insist that the U.S.S.R. remain militantly atheistic and communistic in order to fulfill Lenin's intentions?

We should reject the nebulous doctrine of "original intent" and assert instead the doctrine of "legitimate intent." It matters not whether the Founding Fathers intended to proscribe abortion; what matters is that no government can ever legitimately intend to allow innocent human beings to be murdered by abortion or by any other means.

We must forego dependence on mechanical doctrines such as "original intent," "strict constructionism," and "states' rights," because these mechanical, amoral, manmade concepts are insufficient foundations for launching an effective attack on the grave moral evil of abortion.

"Original intent" and "strict constructionism" would have been workable concepts had the Supreme Court not been commandeered by liberal judicial activists years ago. But "original intent" and "strict constructionism" are hardly the cures for decades of liberal judicial activism: What's needed is a heavy dose of righteous judicial activism to remedy the deadly effects of such artificial concoctions as *Roe v. Wade*. We need to focus on the higher law and we need to argue more from the moral ground of the higher law than from the morally neutral ground of the U.S. Constitution.

The pro-life movement should also re-evaluate its relationship to "conservatism." Conservatism values preservation of the status quo, and the status quo is abortion. Conservatism values amoral, mechanical, and structural solutions to moral problems (i.e., it sees abortion as a states' rights issue rather than as a crime against God and man). Conservatism elevates tradition and form over righteousness and content. Conservatism can be as morally bankrupt as liberalism. The pro-life movement should be careful not to confuse itself with conservatism, and it must not equate pro-life principles with traditional family values. Unfortunate examples of conservatism and traditional family values in America are such things as racism, materialism, xenophobia, and selfishness.

The pro-life movement could also benefit from admitting that God is not a Republican. Yes, the Republican Party has been the party of choice for pro-lifers for about a decade now, and yes, the Democratic Party is pregnant with baby-bashers. But by swearing blind allegiance to one political party, we have nullified our political power.

Pro-lifers have become to the Republican Party what gays have become to the Democratic Party: an embarrassing constituency that is bought cheaply with a few vague, unfulfilled campaign promises that are soon forgotten. We are taken for granted because our support was never really in question.

It is time that pro-lifers admit that we have sold our cause for a bowl of pottage. We have given the Republican Party our unquestioning support because the party talked nicely to us. And worse, we have failed to demand that elected Republican officials undertake effective pro-life initiatives. It is high time that pro-lifers began to demand greater accountability from the Republican Party, and it's time we began to withhold our votes and dollars and support from Republican candidates who fail to demonstrate effective pro-life *action*. Action, not dialogue, not promises, must determine our votes and our support.

The pro-life movement must regain its backbone. We must become relevant, unyielding, uncompromising. We must become radically persistent and persistently radical. And in doing so, we will force the pro-death camps to give up ground, and ultimately, we will see the triumph of good over evil.

State

Pro-lifers in every state must demand accounting from their state governments for how every dollar of Title X and Title XX funds are spent. To what and to whom do the dollars go? How much goes to Planned Parenthood affiliates? What are the state rules? Who administers the programs?

Each state should pass a Truth in Contraception Act requiring all birth control devices and chemicals to contain warnings about incurable venereal diseases (including AIDS and herpes) and disclosing actual in-use reliability factors over extended time periods and prohibiting their sale as "safe sex" enablers. This requirement should extend to (1) birth control devices and chemical labeling, and (2) birth control devices and chemical dispensing, providing that the warning must be posted conspicuously in dispensing locations.

States should de-fund all amoral Planned Parenthood-style comprehensive sex-ed courses. State funding should be limited to chastity-based programs such as *Sex Respect*.

In addition, state legislatures should prohibit state funds from being provided to school districts that offer courses which teach that sex outside of marriage can be safe or responsible, or that promote fornication or homosexuality as legitimate options. Schools should be required to obtain parental permission before instructing children in *any* sex education material, and they must be required to teach sex-ed only in sex-segregated classes, so as not to aggravate peer pressure.

States should also prohibit the use by public schools of any sex-ed materials that are written by, supplied by, or obtained from, any organization that manufactures, sells, distributes, or dispenses contraceptives, that performs abortions, or that charges for sexual counseling.

States should pass a Peer Pressure Reduction Act which would:

1. Prohibit any school from providing abortions or referrals for abortions, or contraceptive counseling or referral; or from dispensing or providing prescriptions for contraceptive chemicals or devices.

2. Instruct all school districts to promote an environment that encourages teen chastity and that devalues teen promiscuity. Schools should be required to formulate programs and provide instruction to encourage teen chastity.

States should also outlaw the dispensing of contraceptives to unmarried minors without parental consent. In addition, we must insist on more vigorous prosecution of incest and statutory rape cases, since it is these few very young (nine-, ten-, eleven-year-old) pregnancies that are so often used as bludgeons to force how-to sex-ed courses on very young children.

We must also work very hard toward passing strong state anti-abortion statutes which specifically state that they become effective to the extent permissible upon any reversal of *Roe v. Wade*.

City

Pro-lifers should investigate city health department and social services or human services agencies to determine any formal or informal ties to Planned Parenthood. Any connections found should be exposed at city council meetings and legislation should be proposed to force the city to disengage itself from Planned Parenthood. Planned Parenthood's racist background and eugenic population targeting should be exposed.

City family planning programs should be barred from using taxpayer funds to dispense nonbarrier contraceptive devices to unmarried people. Also, city agencies (including police, health and social services) should be prohibited from using funds for abortions or referring patients to any organization that performs abortions.

County

County hospitals must be prohibited from performing abortions or referring for abortions. This may be done by budgetary or legislative initiatives. Any formal ties with Planned Parenthood should be exposed and severed.

Schools

We must work toward the removal of traditional, amoral, Planned Parenthood-style contraception-oriented sex indoctrination courses from our schools, and we must implement chastity-based, moral sex education curricula. Where resources are scarce, it is probably better to concentrate on installing good moral sex education curricula in schools that have no sex education, than to undertake intensive battles to try to unseat bad sex education programs.

Clinics

Clinic level activism involves two main processes: information gathering and truth telling. Planned Parenthood is a very large, wealthy, powerful, savvy organization, and it excels at manipulating public opinion through the media. For this reason a thorough information-gathering phase is crucial to a successful truth telling effort.

Information about Planned Parenthood clinics must be obtained directly from the clinics. Institute a regular program of trash collection and analysis. Visit the clinic's dumpster and retrieve its trash. At first, take *all* the trash. After a while, you will learn what kinds of trash to take and what kinds to leave behind; but initially, look at every piece of trash.

Planned Parenthood is likely to yield valuable information on such things as:

- botched abortions
- lawsuits against the clinic
- upcoming media campaigns, banquets, speaking engagements
- ties to elected officials and local schools
- detailed financial data
- names of abortionists and staff members
- minutes of board meetings
- problems peculiar to the clinic

There is no aspect of the clinic's operations that cannot be learned from its trash. This step is crucial.

You should also visit the clinic, talk to the staff, browse through the library. Observe and listen, and remember to write down any pertinent information for later use.

Send clients into the clinic for pregnancy tests and abortion counseling. Find out whether they refer for adoptions, and if so, where. Pick up as much clinic literature as possible.

Send a teen-ager in for contraception and counseling. See if she can obtain contraceptives on government funding, and if so, under what program.

Be sure that you find out the names of the doctors who perform abortions, and of the executive director and staff members who assist in the abortions. You will also need to find their home addresses and the names and locations of their private practices.

The second phase is truth telling. Truth telling involves using the information you obtained to expose and denounce the clinic *and* its employees *and* its board members.

Hold a press conference and denounce the clinic for not providing women with adoption services, for dispensing contraceptives to unmarried minors without parental consent, for abortion-biased counseling, for spreading outdated and dangerous myths about "safe sex," for botching abortions, and the like. Express shock that the clinic receives government funding, and call for an investigation of these abuses by the city or state.

Picket the clinic's board meetings. The clinic's board undoubtedly includes doctors and businessmen (and maybe even some clergymen) who may be pro-choice, but who certainly are not so committed to Planned Parenthood that they are willing tc have their names publicly linked with *baby-killing* or contributing to the delinquency of minors or promoting teen fornication or fostering racial genocide. Businessmen, especially, *hate* bad publicity, and being picketed about abortion or teen fornication or racism is really bad publicity. In other words, it works.

Picketing the private residences of the doctors and of the executive director of the clinic can also be very effective. Clearly identify the doctor by name and address, and leaflet the neighborhood prior to the picket with a handbill identifying the abortionist by name and address and describing how he profits from murdering children.

Picketing can also be effective at Planned Parenthood clinics, but pickets are best designed as specific events. For instance, Planned Parenthood clinics are ripe targets for pickets to expose their complicity in fostering AIDS. Planned Parenthood has consistently portrayed homosexuality as healthy and normal and has promoted and aided teen fornication. In addition, Planned Parenthood has misrepresented birth control as safe (even though *birth* control does not prevent venereal disease transmission) and has alleged condoms to be both safe and effective when they are neither. Planned Parenthood's guilt in fostering and continuing the AIDS crisis needs to be highlighted by high-profile picketing.

The most effective tactic for opposing individual Planned Parenthood clinics, however, is not picketing. The best tactic is sidewalk preaching combined with picketing. Planned Parenthood clinics despise preaching. The truth rattles the workers, unsettles the clients, and brings a general fear and dread and gloom upon the clinic. Consistently applied week-after-week, sidewalk preaching and counseling will always make a difference.

In Houston, consistent sidewalk preaching, applied over a period of two years, resulted in lowered employee morale, an inability to retain good nursing staff, unfavorable media exposure, and an occasional saved baby. But the real dividends were reaped when another local abortuary was commandeered for four hours one Saturday morning by seventy pro-lifers participating in a rescue mission (eighteen were jailed for trespassing; six babies were saved, one of whom was born only two weeks later). Because of the consistent preaching that had been done at the Planned Parenthood clinic prior to the rescue mission, Planned Parenthood never again opened on Saturdays. The clinic was terrified of being invaded by a "rabid" mob of pro-lifers. As a direct result of closing on Saturdays, the Planned Parenthood clinic saw its abortion volume drop by one-third, meaning that sixty babies a month were saved.

Summary

Planned Parenthood is very vulnerable to well-planned opposition efforts because its programs are dismal failures. We need to use a wide variety of legal, educational, and confrontational tactics to resist, expose, and oppose Planned Parenthood's deadly operations.

It is imperative, however, that we do not devote all of our resources merely to trying to thwart some of Planned Parenthood's most destructive campaigns, such as the campaign to install contraceptive-dispensing sex clinics in American schools. We must remember that Planned Parenthood has always maintained a threefold thrust: clinics, schools, and *churches*.

To a large extent, we have already lost the important battles over clinics and schools. Still, we need to continue our efforts in those arenas to halt and then neutralize Planned Parenthood's destructive influence in establishing sex education programs, school-based sex clinics, and abortion chambers. But it is imperative that we devote our greatest energy to solidifying our last remaining beachhead—our presence in churches.

We must make the establishment of moral, life-affirming sex education programs in churches our highest priority. If we continue to neglect our responsibility in this crucial arena, we will soon find ourselves without a forum to offer a sane and healthful alternative to Planned Parenthood's irrational vision of failure and death.

We must work in and with the church to develop programs and organizations that reach teens long before they are drawn into the whole shabby universe of promiscuity and premarital pregnancy and venereal disease and abortion. With the church's help, we can do more than simply oppose Planned Parenthood: we can actively sow seeds of hope and success in people's lives, insuring a better future for our teens, our families, our nation.